NANOMEDICINES

Edited by **Muhammad Akhyar Farrukh**

Nanomedicines

http://dx.doi.org/10.5772/intechopen.71939
Edited by Muhammad Akhyar Farrukh

Part of IntechOpen Book Series: Biomedical Engineering, Volume 5
Book Series Editor: Robert Koprowski

Contributors

Velichka Andonova, Nadezhda Ivanova, Viliana Gugleva, Mirena Dobreva, Stefan Radnev Stefanov, Ivaylo Pehlivanov, Koushlesh Mishra, Chanchal Deep Kaur, Shekhar Verma, Anil Kumar Sahu, Pankaj Kashyap, Sarawati Prasad Mishra, Deepak Kumar Dash, Teodora Mocan, Ofelia Mosteanu, Cristian Tudor Matea, Teodora Atena Pop, Nadim Al Hajjar, Cosmin Puia, Cristina Bura, Lucian Mocan, Luminita Furcea, Rasedee Abdullah, Heshu Rahman, Qiana Matthews, Brennetta Crenshaw, Brian Sims

First published in London, United Kingdom, 2019 by IntechOpen
IntechOpen is the global imprint of INTECHOPEN LIMITED, registered in England and Wales, registration number: 11086078, The Shard, 25th floor, 32 London Bridge Street
London, SE19SG – United Kingdom
Printed in Croatia

British Library Cataloguing-in-Publication Data
A catalogue record for this book is available from the British Library

Additional hard copies can be obtained from orders@intechopen.com

Nanomedicines, Edited by Muhammad Akhyar Farrukh
p. cm.
Print ISBN 978-1-78985-283-7
Online ISBN 978-1-78985-284-4
ISSN: 2631-5343

For EU product safety concerns:
IN TECH d.o.o., Prolaz Marije Krucifikse Kozulić 3, 51000 Rijeka, Croatia,
info@intechopen.com or visit our website at intechopen.com.

IntechOpen Book Series
Biomedical Engineering
Volume 5

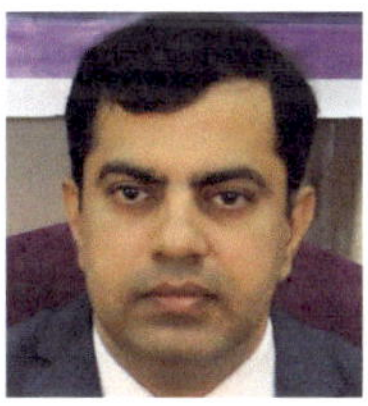

Dr. Muhammad Akhyar Farrukh is currently serving at the Forman Christian College (A Chartered University), Pakistan, as Associate Professor of Chemistry. He has been duly awarded three gold medals for his outstanding academic performance in chemistry and four gold medals for his excellent performance in research and service to society. He has been awarded many international and national awards: Representative of Pakistan by UNESCO in Morocco, Young Chemist Award by IUPAC in Italy, Young Scientist Awards by TWAS in Egypt and IAP/GYA in Germany, Young Scientist Award by IAP/World Economic Forum in China, Young Researcher Award by the Council for Lindau Nobel Laureate Meetings, IUPAC-2015, Award for Chemists as an outstanding chemist from developing countries in South Korea, Research Productivity Awards with Category A, B, and C, Productive Scientist of Pakistan with rank at 11th in Pakistan in Chemistry category Young Scientists in 2017 and 2018, and SATHA Innovation Award 2018 with Gold Medal.

Editor of Volume 5:
Muhammad Akhyar Farrukh
Forman Christian College (A Chartered University), Lahore, Pakistan

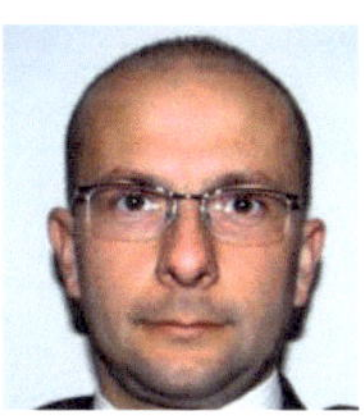

Robert Koprowski, MD (1997), PhD (2003), Habilitation (2015), is a lecturer at the Department of Biomedical Computer Systems, Institute of Computer Science, University of Silesia, Poland. For 20 years, he has been dealing with analysis and processing of biomedical images with a particular emphasis on the full automation of measurement for a large inter-individual variability of patients. He is the author of dozens of papers with an impact factor (IF) and more than a hundred of other papers as well as the author or coauthor of six books. Additionally, he is the author of several national and international patents in the field of biomedical devices and imaging. Since 2011, he has been a reviewer of grants and projects (including EU projects) in the field of biomedical engineering.

Book Series Editor:
Robert Koprowski
University of Silesia, Poland

Contents

Preface

Nanomedicine is the application of nanotechnology (a nanometer is a billionth of a meter) in medicines at an atomic, molecular, and supramolecular level. Nanomedicine covers a wide range of topics from the development of nanomaterials for the use in medicines to the synthesis of nanomedicines with their multiple applications. The major focus of this book is on developments in nanomedicines and their effectiveness compared to conventional drugs.

Some drugs are administered twice daily for days and weeks. However, the frequency of administration and dosage of drug can be reduced to increase patient compliance when prepared at the nanoscale level with polymers. Nanopharmaceutics is also an emerging field and deals with the formation or development of nanodrugs or therapeutic systems at nanoscale level in the range from 1 to 1000 nm.

Nanomaterials such as carbon nanotubes, biodegradable polymers, dendrimers, nanoliposomes, polymeric micelles, metallic nanoparticles, polymeric nanoparticles, etc. are used in drug formulations. Many factors are considered very important during the synthesis of nanomedicines such as particle size, releasing profile of a drug from the polymer, shelf life and absorption and distribution rate, stability and storage conditions, etc.

This book contains five chapters from leading scientists working in the area of nanomedicines. Particular topics that are highlighted are exosomes, nanoantimicrobial solutions, transethosomes, nanoethosomes, nanoparticles, multifunctional drugs, and natural dietary products.

Exosomes are nanosized vesicles enriched in enzymes, heat shock proteins, membrane trafficking proteins, etc. and are used as potential carriers for therapeutics, biomarkers for diagnosis of various diseases that are associated with cancer, genetics, viruses, bacteria, parasites, etc. Transethosomes and nanoethosomes are employed to overcome the challenge associated with the vesicular system, having better skin permeation of bioactive agents. Information on methods of preparation, characterization, and pharmaceutical uses of nanoethosomes and transethosomes is presented in this book.

Infectious diseases associated with intracellular bacteria are important public health concerns and are a major threat to the worldwide medical community. An overview of intracellular compartments where bacteria can reside and deliberate how nanomedicines have the potential to enhance intracellular disease therapy, sustained drug release, and drug delivery to intracellular locations harboring bacteria is given in detail.

Physicochemical characteristics and antibacterial and anticancer properties, which silver nanoparticles obtained by plant-mediated methods, and their application as drug delivery systems with a critical view on the possible toxicity on the human body are also very important topics to be considered. It is established that a diet rich in fresh fruits, vegetables, seeds, grains and legumes, and antioxidants may help prevent various human diseases. However, diet is not a cure for the treatment of severe diseases. Drugs with poor solubility encounter limited transport during oral administration because of low concentration gradient between the gut and blood vessels. New delivery methods need to be developed using natural dietary plant metabolites to increase the body fluid saturation solubility of poorly soluble drugs, which is explained in this book.

I would like to thank Author Service Manager Ms. Jasna Bozic for her cooperation throughout the process of the publication of this book.

Dr. Muhammad Akhyar Farrukh
Associate Professor
Department of Chemistry
Forman Christian College (A Chartered University)
Lahore, Pakistan

Chapter 1

Biological Function of Exosomes as Diagnostic Markers and Therapeutic Delivery Vehicles in Carcinogenesis and Infectious Diseases

Brennetta J. Crenshaw, Brian Sims and
Qiana L. Matthews

Additional information is available at the end of the chapter

http://dx.doi.org/10.5772/intechopen.80225

Abstract

Exosomes are nano-sized vesicles that are formed during inward budding of multivesicular bodies and the maturation of endosomes. They are secreted by almost all cell types under normal, pathological, and physiological conditions. They are found in mostly all biological fluids, such as breast milk, blood, urine, and semen. Exosomes are involved in cell-to-cell communication through the biological transfer of lipids, proteins, DNAs, RNAs, mRNAs, and miRNAs. Exosomes are enriched in tetraspanins, enzymes, heat shock proteins, and membrane trafficking proteins. There are numerous techniques that are used to isolate, purify, and characterize exosomes from biofluids. Isolation/purification techniques include ultracentrifugation, filtration, sucrose density gradient centrifugation, etc. Characterization techniques include flow cytometry, electron microscopy, NanoSight tracking analysis, Western blot, etc. These techniques are often used to help principal investigators understand the properties and biological functions of exosomes. However, some of these techniques can be very complicated and challenging, resulting in various drawbacks. Exosomes can be used as potential carriers for therapeutics. Thus, they can serve as biomarkers to diagnosis various diseases that are associated with cancer, genetics, viruses, bacteria, parasites, etc. Therefore, with advances in science and technology, many innovative techniques have been established to exploit the biological properties of exosomes.

Keywords: exosome, extracellular vesicles, biogenesis, therapeutics, cancer, infectious diseases, drug delivery

1. The discovery of exosomes

In the early 1980s, researchers Pan, Stahl, and Johnstone discovered a complex mode of extracellular vesicle (EV) secretion while studying the loss of transferrin during the maturation of reticulocytes in blood [1–4]. EVs were believed to bud directly from plasma membrane fragments that were isolated from cultured cells and human bodily fluids [1, 2, 5–7]. The research group showed that small vesicles were formed by inward budding inside an intracellular endosome which lead to the formation of multivesicular bodies (MVBs) [1, 8–10]. The MVBs produce intraluminal vesicles (ILVs) and fuse with the plasma membrane, releasing their contents into the extracellular environment [1, 8, 9]. The ILVs were termed "exosomes" in the late 1980s by Johnstone [2, 9]. Since their discovery approximately 40 years ago [3, 4, 8], exosomes have gained tremendous attention due to their involvement in intercellular communication [11]. EVs were originally believed to be waste products of the cell [8, 12, 13]. We currently recognize EVs as much more.

2. Exosome biogenesis and secretion

Exosomes are generated in the endosomal membrane when the ILVs of MVBs are formed during the maturation of early and late endosomes [1]. During maturation, MVBs are fated for lysosomal degradation or fused with the plasma membrane which leads to the secretion of ILVs as exosomes [1, 14]. The generation of the ILVs in MVBs contains the lateral segregation of cargo at the endosomal limiting membrane [15, 16]. In addition, it involves the formation of an inward budding vesicle and the release in the endosomal lumen of the membrane vesicle containing a small portion of cytosol [15, 16].

The Endosomal Sorting Complex Responsible for Transport (ESCRT) mediates exosome biogenesis [1, 17–19]. ESCRTs consist of approximately 20 proteins that are divided into the ESCRT-0, -I, -II, and –III complexes [20, 21]. These complexes contain ubiquitin-binding subunits [18, 21, 22]. The ESCRT-0 complex identifies and sequentially binds to ubiquitylated proteins in the endosomal membrane [23]. The ESCRT-I and -II complexes are responsible for membrane deformation into buds with sequential cargo [21]. The ESCRT-III complex drives vesicle scission [21, 24].

ESCRT-0 contains the hepatocyte growth factor-regulated tyrosine kinase substrate (HRS) protein [22]. HRS identifies ubiquitylated cargo proteins and other constituents in a complex that consist of clathrin, the epidermal growth factor receptor pathway substrate 15 gene, and signal-transducing adaptor molecule [18, 25]. Most importantly, HRS recruit tumor susceptibility gene 101 of the ESCRT-I complex [26]. ESCRT-I is then involved in the recruitment of ESCRT-III, through ESCRT-II or the ESCRT-accessory protein ALG-2 interacting protein-X (Alix) [26]. Lastly, the separation and recycling of the ESCRT machinery interacts with the AAA-ATPase vacuolar protein sorting 4 [19, 27].

Exosomes are secreted by many cell types during normal, physiological, and pathological conditions [14, 28, 29]. They are secreted from cancer cells [28, 30], platelets [31], neurons

[32], epithelial cells [28, 33, 34], dendritic cells [28, 35], B and T cells [28, 36], astrocytes [28, 37], endothelial cells [28, 38], mast cells [31, 39], and mesenchymal stem cells [28, 40]. Also, exosomes have been identified in most bodily fluids, such as nasal secretion [28, 41], blood [42], serum [28, 43], ascites [44], amniotic fluid [44], urine [28, 45], breast milk [28, 46], and saliva [28, 43].

Depending on the cell type, exosomes are mainly secreted by the constitutive release pathway and/or inducible release pathway [28, 47–51]. In the constitutive secretion pathway, proteins are sorted into vesicles in the Golgi and transported to the cell surface where they fuse with the plasma membrane via exocytosis. In addition, Rab guanosine triphosphatases (GTPases) [52, 53], hetrotrimeric G-protein [52], protein kinase D [52, 54], glycosphingolipids, and flotillin [52] are involved in this pathway. Specifically, several Rab GTPases have been shown to act as key regulators of the exosome secretory pathway [49]. Rabs are a large group of small GTPases that regulate protein transport via endocytic and exocytic pathways in all cell types [52, 55]. In addition, Rabs are involved in membrane trafficking (i.e. vesicle budding, membrane fusion, and the transport of vesicles along actin and tubulin) [53]. Rab GTPases are composed of approximately 70 distinct proteins [56, 57]. Common Rab proteins include Rab11, Rab27, and Rab35 [58, 59]. These proteins are all involved in the transport of endolysosomal vesicles toward the plasma membrane [60].

Rab11 was the first Rab GTPase reported study that involved exosome secretion in human leukemic K562 cells by Savina et al. [61, 62]. Specifically, Rab11 is involved in the recycling from an endosomal compartment to the plasma membrane [63–65]. Both Rab27a and Rab 27b function in MVE docking at the plasma membrane in several cancer cell lines *in vivo* and *in vitro* [49, 55, 66]. Rab35 mediates MVB docking or tethering in oligodendroglia cells as reported by Hsu et al.[58, 61]. They revealed that the inhibition of Rab35 leads to intracellular accumulation of endosomal vesicles and impairs exosome secretion [58, 61]. In addition, Hsu et al. showed that Rab35 localizes to the surface of oligodendroglia in a GTP-dependent manner, where it regulates vesicular density [58, 61].

Inducible secretion is regulated by many cellular processes [67–69]. This pathway is regulated by stimuli, such as heat shock, hypoxia [52], DNA damage [52, 67, 70], increased intracellular calcium release [52, 67, 70], thrombin [52], extracellular ATP [52, 67], and lipopolysaccharide 39 stimulation [35, 52]. In 2012, King et al. demonstrated that the release of exosomes in breast cancer cells is promoted by hypoxia [71]. In addition, they demonstrated the hypoxic response could potentially be mediated by the hypoxia-inducible factor-1α—a group of transcription factors that are targeted for degradation under normal oxygen conditions by the action of specific O_2–, iron- and 2-oxoglutarate dependent prolyl hydroxylases [71, 72]. Another study was reported by Hooper and colleagues in 2012 [73]. In their study, they investigated the inducible release of exosomes cultured from rat microglia cells treated with recombinant carrier-free Wnt3a protein- a family of cysteine rich glycoproteins that play a role in tumorigenesis and act as morphogens during development [69, 73]. They observed that these Wnt3-induced cells increased exosome secretion through a glycogen synthase kinase 3-independent mechanism [73]. The process of exosome biogenesis and secretion is summarized in **Figure 1**.

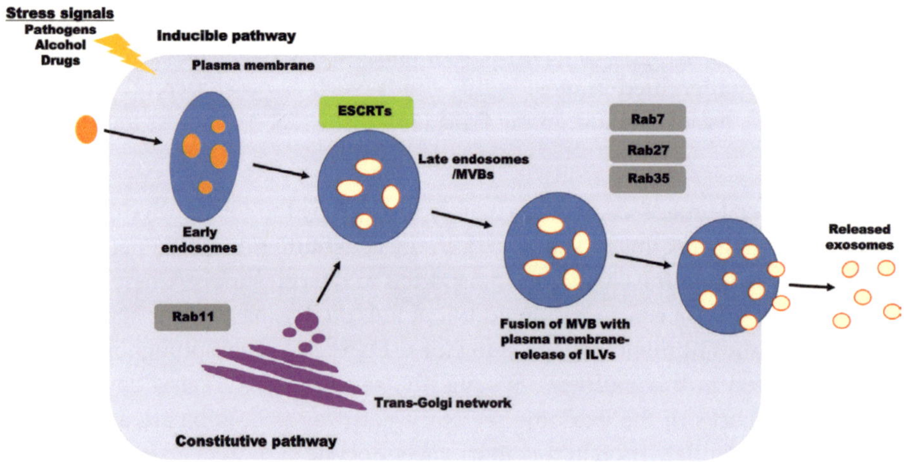

Figure 1. Biogenesis and secretion of exosomes. Exosome biogenesis and secretion is a complex process. Exosome secretion can occur by two different mechanisms, constitutive or inducible secretion. One or both of these pathways maybe operational depending on the condition of the cell. Constitutive exosome secretion occurs in various cell types under normal physiological and pathological conditions. Inducible exosome secretion is regulated by stressors (e.g. pathogens, alcohol, drugs). Multivesicular bodies (MBVs), intraluminal vesicles (ILVs), Trans-Golgi network and the Endosomal Sorting Complex Responsible for Transport (ESCRT) are four important compartments involved in exosome biogenesis and secretion. Rab guanosine triphosphatases (GTPases) (7, 11, 27, 35 etc.) are also depicted, they play an important role in exosome secretion.

3. Composition of exosomes

Exosomes carry a group of specific proteins, lipids, RNA, microRNA (miRNA), and DNAs, that represents their cells of origin [28, 56, 74], as depicted in **Figure 2**. Recent studies have shown that exosomes contain approximately 194 lipids, 4563 proteins, 1639 messenger RNAs (mRNAs), and 764 miRNAs [28, 75–77]. Exosomes are enriched in molecules, such as the major histocompatibility molecules (MHC) class I and II that play a key role in immunoregulation by processing antigenic peptides [28, 78]. Also, exosomes contain tetraspanins that serve as unique markers [79]. Tetraspanins include: cluster of differentiation (CD) 9, CD63, CD81, and CD82, as well as adhesion molecules CD54 and CD11b [26, 28, 78]. In addition, exosomes are enriched with heat shock proteins (hsps) which act as chaperones and play a key role in cellular responses that are associated with environmental stress. Hsps assist with protein folding and trafficking. Common exosomal proteins include Hsp60, Hsp70, Hsp90, and heat shock protein cognate 70 [16, 78]. Along with tetraspanins and hsps, exosomes contain cytoplasmic proteins such as Rabs and annexins [26, 61]. These proteins promote the fusion of MVB with the cell membrane and the removal of exosomes. Clathrin, Alix, Tumor susceptibility gene 101 (TSG) 101), and ubiquitin are exosomal constituents that are involved in the biogenesis of MVBs [78]. Enzymes that makeup the composition of exosomes consist of protein kinase G (PKG), ATPase, Glyceraldehyde 3-phosphate dehydrogenase (GAPDH), and enolase. Signal transduction proteins, ADP-ribosylation factor (ARF) 1, cell division control protein 42 (CDC42), epidermal growth factor receptor (EGFR), β-catenin, guanine nucleotide-binding G proteins (G proteins), phosphatidylinositol 3-kinase (P13K), mucin 1 (MUC 1), 14-3-3, and syntenin [68, 78, 80]. Viral proteins, such as group-specific antigen (Gag), Human immunodeficiency virus negative regulatory factor (HIV Nef), Herpes simplex virus glycoprotein B

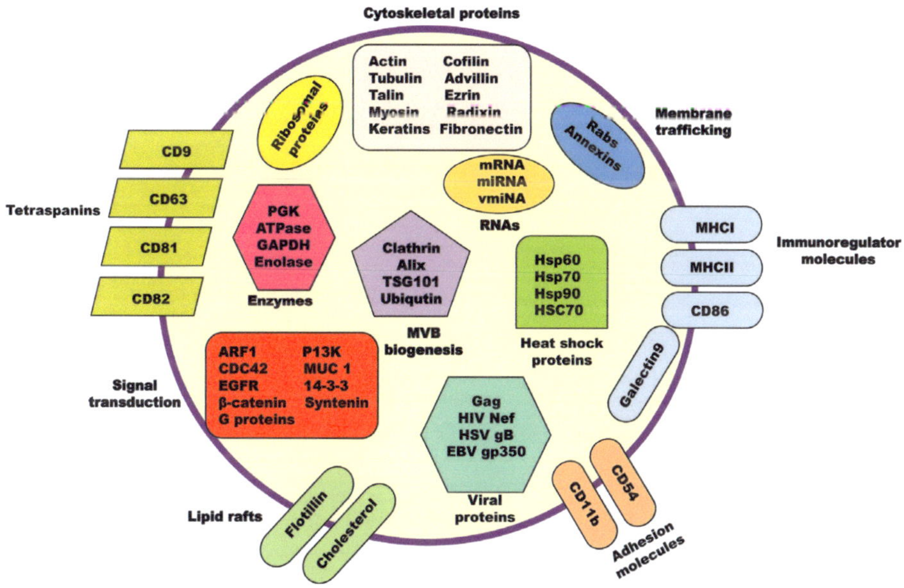

Figure 2. Composition of exosomes. Proteomic, Biochemical, and Immunological investigations have identified many specific proteins and RNAs present in some exosomes. This is a limited representation of common molecules present within some exosomes. Molecules illustrated here are grouped based on category function or protein class: Tetraspanins, Cytoskeletal proteins, Membrane trafficking proteins, Immunoregulator molecules, Adhesion molecules, Lipid rafts, Signal transduction molecules, viral proteins and RNAs.

(HSV gB), Epstein–Barr virus (EBV) gp350 also make up the composition of some exosomes [78, 81]. Exosomes that contain RNA can serve as an alternate pathway of cellular communication [82, 83]. Thus, mRNAs that are found in exosomes can be transferred to target cells and translated into proteins [84]. miRNAs, such as miR-1, miR-15, miR-16, miR-151, miR-375, and lethal-7 play a role in hematopoiesis, exocytosis, tumorigenesis, and angiogenesis [28, 85, 86].

4. Exosome isolation/purification methods

Exosomes are isolated from a wide spectrum of biological fluids [87, 88]. To examine the quality of isolated exosomes, numerous methods have been developed to examine and measure their morphology, composition, quantity, and size distribution [88, 89]. With advances in science and technology, many innovative techniques have been established to exploit a specific trait of exosomes, such as their size, shape, density, and surface proteins to aid in their isolation and purification [88, 90]. However, each method has advantages and disadvantages as shown in **Table 1**.

4.1. Ultracentrifugation and filtration-based exosome isolation

Ultracentrifugation is a centrifugation process used for generating acceleration up to 100,000 × g (approx. 9800 km/s^2) [88]. Differential ultracentrifugation is often used to isolate exosomes [88, 91]. The isolation of exosomes by differential ultracentrifugation contains numerous centrifugation steps, which uses centrifugal force to get rid of residual cells, cellular

Isolation/purification methods	Mechanism	Advantages	Disadvantages
Differential ultracentrifugation [79, 91]	Remove residual cells, large vesicles, and cellular debris; precipitate exosomes [79]	Standard method used to isolate exosomes from cultured media and biological fluids [79, 91]	Effectiveness of the method is lower when biological fluids are used for analysis [79] co-precipitation of protein aggregates, apoptotic bodies, or nucleosomal fragments, which may lead to less sample purity and less correctly bound proteins [91]
Sucrose gradient centrifugation [91]	Separate vesicles based on their different flotation densities [91, 97]	Allows separation of the low-density exosomes from other vesicles, particles and contaminants [91]	Cannot separate exosomes from viruses because of their similarities in density and size [91]
Filtration [79, 91]	Used to separate exosomes from proteins and other macroparticles using ultrafiltration membranes [79]	Allows separation of soluble molecules and small particles from exosomes [79]	Loss of analysis due to adhesion. Contamination of isolated EVs. Exosomes can potentially be deformed or damaged due to additional force being applied pass the analyzed liquid through the membrane [79, 91]
Size exclusion chromatography [79]	Applies a column packed with porous polymeric beads which separates the particles based on their size [79]	Allows precise separation of large and small molecules and application of various solutions. Compared to centrifugation methods, the structure of exosomes isolated by chromatography is not affected by shearing force [79]	Requires a long running time, which limits applications of chromatographical isolation for processing multiple biological samples [79]
Microfluidics [91]	Microscale isolation based on a variety of properties of exosomes like immunoaffinity, size, and density [91]	Energy efficient, portable, fast processing time, low cost, easy automation and integration [91]	Lack of standardization and large scale tests on clinical samples, lack of method validation, moderate to low sample capacity [91]
ExoQuick™ [91, 111]	Precipitates exosomes overnight through incubation [91, 111]	Fast and easy processing; additional equipment is not needed for isolation [91, 111]	Lack specificity toward exosomes; biological fluids are difficult to resuspend [91, 111]

Table 1. Advantages and disadvantages of isolation/purification methods.

debris, and large vesicles [79, 88]. In addition, these steps are used to precipitate exosomes [79, 88]. There are various protocols available for this isolation technique. First, cell culture is subjected to a low speed centrifugation using a Sorvall RT600 centrifuge with a swinging bucket rotor (Thermo Fisher Scientific). This is applied to remove cells and apoptotic debris [92, 93]. Next, a higher speed is used to administer and eliminate larger vesicles, whereas, the remaining media is re-suspended in phosphate buffered saline. Lastly, a high speed of centrifugation using a SW41T1 swinging rotor in a Beckman Coulter (Brea, CA, USA) (Optima L-70 K ultracentrifuge) is performed to precipitate exosomes; and the exosome pellet is stored at −80°C until further use [92].

Filtration is a size-based technique that is often used in combination with ultracentrifugation, as depicted in **Figure 3**, for the isolation of exosomes in *in vitro* studies [92–94]. Depending on the size of vesicles, filtration is applied to separate exosomes from proteins and other particles [79]. Filtration membranes that have pore sizes of 0.22, 0.45, or 0.8 μm can be used to collect EVs that are larger than 150 nm [79]. Although filtration is a quick isolation method, it faces challenges, such as contamination of isolated EVs, trapping of EVs in nano or micro pores, and co-purifying abundant proteins EVs isolation [91]. Because of these disadvantages, the maximal recovery of EVs for isolation must be optimized [91].

4.2. Sucrose density gradient centrifugation

Sucrose density gradient centrifugation is a form of centrifugation that is used to measure the density of exosomes in a sucrose gradient [95]. Exosomes have floatation densities ranging from 1.08 to 1.22 g/ml on continuous sucrose gradients [91, 96, 97]. Vesicles that are purified from the Golgi float at 1.05 to 1.12 g/ml; and vesicles that are purified from the endoplasmic reticulum float at 1.18 to 1.25 g/ml [95]. Sucrose density gradient is formed by overlapping lower concentrations of sucrose on higher concentrations in a centrifuge tube. For instance, a sucrose gradient may contain layers ranging from 70% sucrose to 20% sucrose in 10% increments [91, 96, 97]. Since exosomes are generally spread among 3 to 5 segments of the sucrose gradient, it is recommended to perform this separation approximately 5 times the amount of exosomal proteins that is needed to detect exosomes.

4.3. Size exclusion chromatography

Size exclusion chromatography (SEC) is used to separate macroparticles based on size, not molecular weight [79]. Currently, SEC is used to isolate exosomes that are present in urine [98] and blood [79, 99]. This method utilizes a column packed with porous polymeric beads

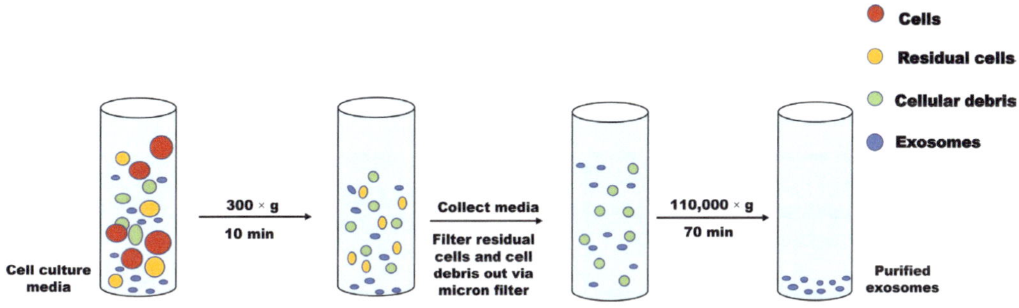

Figure 3. Schematic illustration of differential ultracentrifugation. Cell culture media is collected and centrifuged by means of low speed centrifugation followed by collection of media and filtration using a 0.22-micron filter. The media then undergoes ultracentrifugation pelleting the exosomes which are resuspended in buffer for further use.

that contains several pores and tunnels. In SEC, particles pass through the beads depending on their diameter. Particles that contain small hydrodynamic radii can pass through the pores, hence resulting in late elution [88]. However, particles that contain large hydrodynamic radii, are excluded from entering the pores [88, 100].Correspondingly, SEC is used in combination with ultracentrifugation to isolate/purify exosomes [88, 101]. Rood et al. 2010 demonstrated that ultracentrifugation followed by SEC, significantly enriched urinary exosomes compared to exosomes that were obtained by ultrafiltration or ultracentrifugation alone [101, 102].

4.4. Microfluidics

Microfluidics is the study and manipulation of fluids at the microscale level by means of frictional forces [91, 103]. Microfluidic devices bind specific EVs to antibody-coated surfaces [104, 105]. The EV sample is loaded on a pump that slowly pushes the fluid through the chip. Microfluidic-based technologies ensure that fluid pressure is converted to high shear forces more consistent and efficient than other technologies. By maintaining constant pressure, microfluidic homogenizers ensure that the samples receive the same treatment. As fluids are forced at controlled temperatures and constant pressures through the interaction chamber, particles

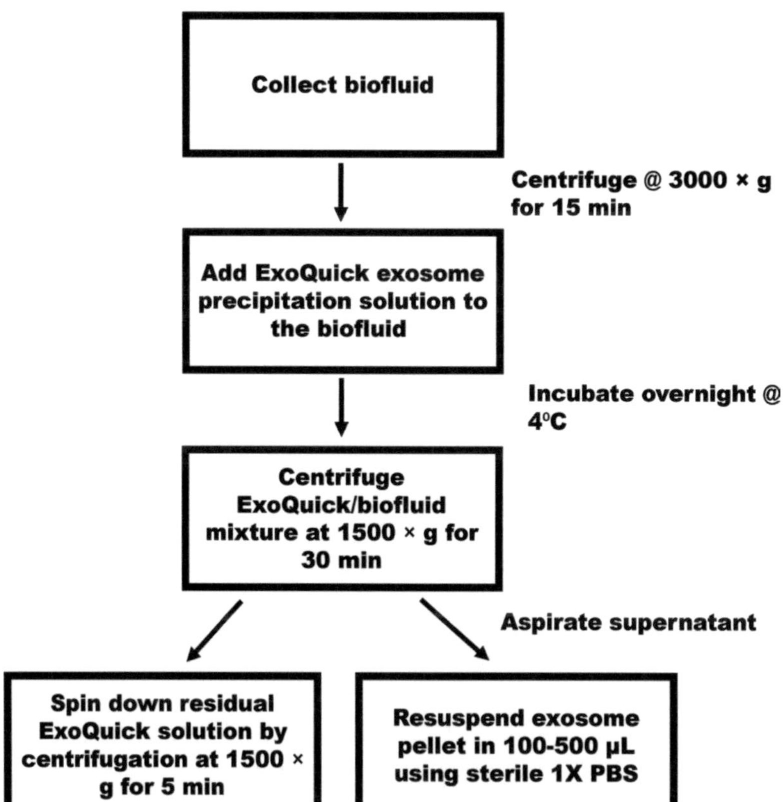

Figure 4. Standard ExoQuick™ protocol. Exosomes are collected be means of several centrifugation and precipitation steps.

experience extremely high shear forces. As a result of these forces, particle size is reduced and particle size distribution curves are constricted. Advantages of this technique include a reduction in processing times, energy consumption, volumes of sample, and material costs [106, 107].

4.5. ExoQuick™

Commercial kits utilizing polyethylene glycol for isolation of exosomes are frequently used in research studies [108–110]. ExoQuick™ (System Biosciences, Mountain View, CA, USA) is the most commonly used kit [108]. This kit is quick and easy to perform, and additional equipment is not necessary for isolation. ExoQuick is a proprietary polymer that can be used to isolate exosomes for a variety of applications, including functional studies (i.e. cell-to-cell signaling), exosomal proteomics, biomarker studies, biology studies (i.e. tumorigenesis), exosomal miRNA profiling, and exosomal metabolomics/lipidomics [111–113]. With the ExoQuick, a mix is added to the samples and the EVs precipitate via incubation overnight. Recent studies have revealed that the highest yield of exosomes was obtained using a combination of ExoQuick with ultracentrifugation [91, 114, 115]. However, contamination of exosomal isolates with non-exosomal materials remains a concern for polymer-based isolation procedures. Furthermore, the polymer substance that is present in the isolate may affect the down-stream analysis [79]. A detailed protocol utilizing ExoQuick is depicted in **Figure 4**.

5. Exosome characterization methods

There are several common techniques that are used to determine the quantity, morphology, and size of exosomes following purification. Exosomes can be characterized using the following techniques: flow cytometry [116], electron microscopy (EM) [117], NanoSight tracking analysis (NTA) [92, 117, 118], Raman spectroscopy (RS) [119], Western blot (WB) [42, 92, 120], and/or ExoCarta database [117, 121].

Flow cytometry is one of the most commonly used techniques used to detect the origin, size, and morphology of circulating EVs [116, 121]. It is a high-throughput, multi-parametric technique that quickly analyzes and quantitates thousands of single cells or particles [121, 122]. In this method, a laser beam with a specific wavelength is directed through a stream of a sheath fluid that contains suspended particles [117]. Next, the emitted scatter and fluorescence is captured and measured by detectors [121]. Due to their small diameter (≤200 nm), detecting, capturing, and examining exosomes is difficult to characterize via flow cytometry [123]. However, proteins that are located on the surface of exosomes can be stained with fluorochrome-conjugated antibodies [124].

EM is often used to characterize and visualize exosomes due their small size [117, 120]. EM uses a beam of electrons to generate an image of the EVs' sample [117]. Electron beams are passed through the sample [117]. The electrons are collected and magnified using special lenses [117]. Typical morphological characteristics of exosomes are spherical shaped and range approximately 30–100 nm [120]. When used in conjunction with immuno-labeling, the surface proteins of exosomes can be determined via electron microscopy [125].

NTA measures the concentration and size distribution of exosomes [92, 117, 126, 127]. An NTA device is composed of a laser light scattering microscope connected to a sensitive charge-coupled device camera, a complementary metal–oxide–semiconductor camera, a hydraulic pump, a measuring chamber, and an analytical software [117, 121]. The hydraulic pump injects particles into the measuring chamber at a fixed flow rate and exposes them to a narrow laser beam [117]. Next, the movement of the illuminated particles is recorded by the complementary metal-oxide-semiconductor [117]. The NTA software then identifies and tracks individual ECVs moving under Brownian motion and relates the movement to a particle size based on the Stokes-Einstein equation [128]:

$$(x, y)^2 = 2\,k^B\,T/3\,r_h\,\pi\eta \tag{1}$$

Figure 5 depicts a graphic representation of the NTA.

RS is a quantitative technique that provides the chemical structure of exosomes based on the illumination of analyzed samples by laser light [129]. It is used to study rotational, vibrational, and other low-frequency transitions in a system [130]. Thus, it provides molecular fingerprints of the samples and enables monitoring of changes that occur in the molecular bond structures [117]. In this method, photons interact with other photons, molecular vibrations, and other excitations in the system. This interaction leads to a slight up or down shift of their energy. The shift in energy provides information about the vibrational transitions in the molecules [121, 130, 131]. Because of these measurements, the chemical composition of single EVs can be obtained [117, 131, 132].

WB is often used to show and confirm the presence of exosomal proteins and specific surface markers [133–135]. Specific surface markers include MHC I and MHC II, tetraspanins CD9, CD63, CD81, Hsp70 and Hsp90, etc. After EVs are isolated, they are lysed. Following lysis, the proteins are separated and analyzed [133]. Although WB is used to identify and confirm the presence of exosomal proteins, it cannot determine the presence of EVs alone. However, WB can be used to identify proteins in purified exosomal samples [120, 133].

Also, to help investigators validate and/or characterize their findings related to exosomes, researchers can use ExoCarta (http://www.exocarta.org/) [136]. ExoCarta is an online database that allows principal investigators the ability to identify and characterize exosomal cargos. The database contains detailed information about lipids, proteins, and RNA sequences that have been identified in specific exosomal preparations [77].

There are many other methods/techniques that are used to detect, identify, visualize, and characterize EVs. Additional techniques that have been used include: Sodium dodecyl sulfate polyacrylamide gel electrophoresis (SDS PAGE) [137], Bradford assay [133], Enzyme-linked immunosorbent assay (ELISA) [133], dynamic light scattering (DLS) [117], mass spectrometry [137, 138], atomic force microscopy (AFM) [139], field-flow fractionation [140], and resistive pulse sensing [141]. Briefly, SDS PAGE, the Bradford assay, and ELISA are used to validate the presence of proteins. In this context, these assays could be used to confirm proteins on exosomes and/or proteins located within exosomes. Whereas, mass spectrometry, AFM, field-flow fractionation, and sensitive pulse sensing is to observe the molecular and physiochemical properties of EVs. These assays are often used to examine,

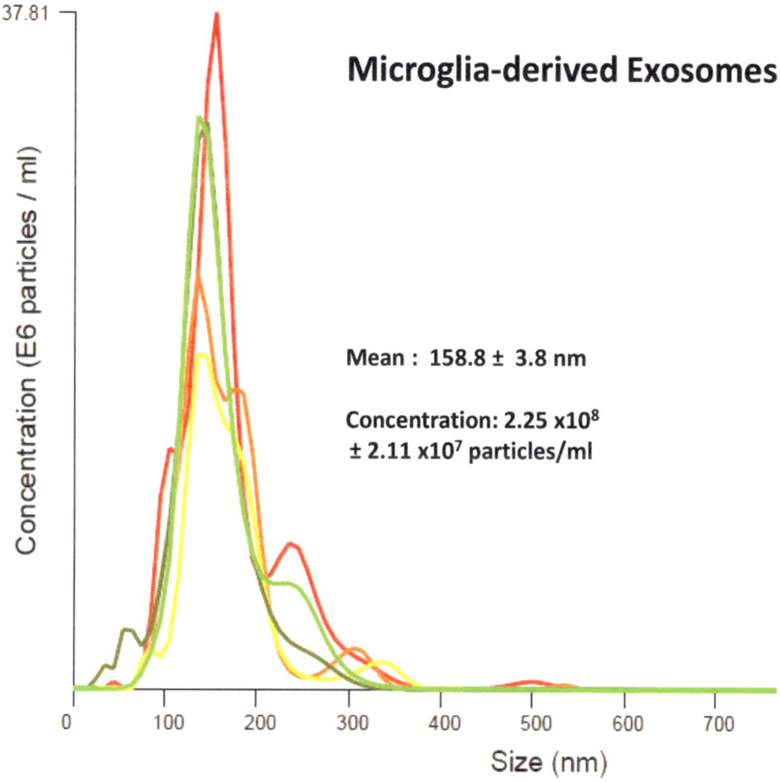

Figure 5. Representation of exosomes by NanoSight tracking analysis (NTA). Microglia-derived exosomes were generated as described in **Figure 3** and confirmed by NTA. In brief, we used the NanoSight LM10 (Malvern Instruments, Inc., Malvern, UK) and NTA v2.0 software to characterize mouse microglia-derived exosomes. All data were collected using five frames and in triplicate. Samples were diluted 1:1000 prior to tracking.

identify, and determine particle size and particle size distribution. Whenever applicable, statistical analyses should be performed to check results found from all methodologies. These analyses could include but are not limited to, Student T-test and analysis of variance (ANOVA).

6. Exosomes in cancer

Exosomes released from cancer cells may impact the cancer microenvironment significantly and alter the fate of proximal cells. These exosomes can mediate intracellular communication between other cancer cells, neighboring stromal cells, and immune cells [142–144]. In 2014, Boelens and team revealed that exosomes can be transferred from stromal cells to breast cancer cells [144, 145]. Due to this transfer, the antiviral retinoic acid-inducible gene 1 enzyme signaling can be activated to regulate the development of therapy-resistance tumor-initiating cells [144, 145]. Several studies have reported that cancer-derived exosomes play a major role in drug resistance, metastasis, angiogenesis, tumorigenesis, tumor growth, and tumor immune escape, as depicted in **Figure 6** [144, 146, 147].

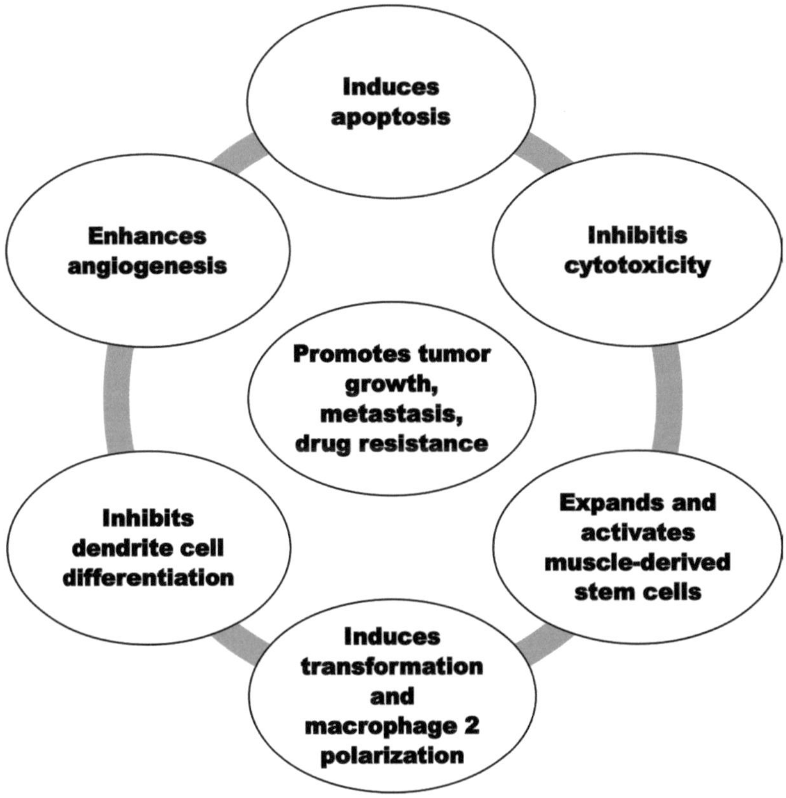

Figure 6. Roles of exosomes in cancer. The multifaceted role of exosomes in carcinogenesis.

6.1. Drug resistance

Resistances to chemotherapy, radiation, or targeted therapies are significant challenges in the treatment of various cancers [148–150]. Recently, it has been demonstrated that exosomes aid in resistance through the transfer of lipids, proteins, mRNAs, and miRNAs [80, 151], which can influence the response to anticancer drugs [152]. Corcoran et al. [153] evaluated the enhancement of exosome secretion by Docetaxel-resistance in prostate cancer. They observed that this enhancement of exosome secretion is due to docetaxel efflux through exosomes [153]. Akao et al. [154] observed that the secretion of tumor-suppressors miRs-145 and miR-34 via exosomes increased 5-fluorouracil resistance in colon cancer cells.

6.2. Metastasis, angiogenesis, and tumorigenesis

It is believed that exosomes mediate signaling in cancer metastasis [155–158]. Exosomes can function as escape routes for miRNAs and proteins that serve as promoters of metastatic pathways. The uptake of exosomes by endothelial cells can stimulate angiogenesis [144, 159, 160]. Grange et al. [159] investigated the role of angiogenesis in renal cell-derived exosomes in lung cancer ascites. Exosomes that are stimulated by hypoxia and heparanase- an enzyme that acts at the cell surface and within the extracellular matrix to degrade heparan sulfate molecules, are associated with angiogenesis of breast cancer, which is the most significant part of breast cancer tumorigenesis [145, 149]. Tumorigenesis is the process that occurs when normal healthy cells transform into cancerous cells. During this process, these cells can secrete exosomes [146, 147]. Several studies have reported that neoplastic transformation of adipose-derived stem cells was induced in response to prostate cancer-derived exosomes [146, 161]. Also, studies have reported that these exosomes deliver mRNA molecules and oncogenic proteins to recipient cells; which subsequently induced tumor formation [146, 162].

6.3. Tumor growth and tumor immune escape

Tumor cells secrete many exosomes [163–166]. Supporting evidence has shown that exosomes released from tumors promote the formation of tumor blood vessels that support tumor growth and extension [144, 146, 149]. Glioblastoma multiforme cell-derived exosomes have been proposed to promote tumor growth by transporting RNA into recipient cells in the microenvironment [142, 143]. In 2011, Kogure and colleagues showed that hepatocellular carcinoma-derived exosomes can modify the transforming growth factor-β-activated kinase 1 expression and associated signaling pathways to augment cell growth in recipient cells [144, 167].

Cancer cells utilize exosomes that contain proteins and nucleic acids to enact an immune escape [144]. It has been shown that they activate dendritic cells, thus priming the immune system to identify and kill cancer cells [168]. Remarkably, exosomes secreted by cancer cells have been proven to express tumor antigens, as well as immune suppressive molecules, such as Fas ligand and Programmed death-ligand 1 [169]. Taken together, these data suggest that cancer cells use exosomes to further advancement of its tumorigenesis.

7. Exosomes in genetic-related diseases

Many types of cells (i.e. neurons, astrocytes, oligodendrocytes, glial) in the central nervous system secret exosomes [32, 170–172]. Exosomes have been reported to aid in the spread of pathological proteins that are involved in neurodegenerative diseases, such as Alzheimer disease (AD) [170, 173], Parkinson's disease (PD) [171, 173, 174] prion diseases [32, 173] and Huntington's disease (HD) [32]. Current studies have shown that exosomes can spread pathological misfolded proteins, which leads to the onset and propagation of AD [170, 173]. AD is the most common form of dementia and characterized by amyloid plaques and neurofibrillary tangles [170, 173]. Accumulating evidence has demonstrated that exosomes play a controversial role in the pathogenesis of Alzheimer [170, 173, 175]. Yuyama et al. [176] observed the presence of exosome-associated amyloid-ß peptide in the cerebrospinal fluid of cynomolgus monkeys and amyloid precursor protein transgenic mice. They concluded that these findings could potentially contribute to AD pathogenesis [176].

Many studies have revealed that exosomes derived from the central nervous system occur in the cerebrospinal fluid and peripheral body fluids, and their contents are altered during disease, making them an appealing target for biomarker development in PD [171, 174]. PD is a disorder that occurs due to the loss of dopamine produced in the brain affecting movement of the body [172, 177]. Exosomes may aid in the spread of toxic α-synuclein protein between cells and induce apoptosis, which could potentially be proposed as a key mechanism underlying the spread of α-synuclein aggregates in the brain and the acceleration of pathology in PD [171, 178]. Comparative studies have shown that the expression of the PD-associated protein α-synuclein is targeted by miR-7 and miR-153 [179–181].

Prion diseases also known as transmissible spongiform encephalopathies are a group of infectious neurodegenerative disorders that affects animals and humans [172, 182]. These diseases are caused by abnormally shaped proteins called prions [177]. Exosome-mediated propagation in prion diseases was reported in 2004 by Fevrier et al. [183, 184]. They observed that the prion protein (PrP)-expressing cells could release normal PrP^{C} and abnormal PrP^{Sc} in association with exosomes [183, 184]. The first reported *in vivo* study related to prion disease pathogenesis was demonstrated 4 years later by Vella et al. 2008 [183, 185]. They revealed PrPC was associated with extracellular vesicles that were found in the CSF of sheep [183, 185].

HD is a hereditary neurodegenerative disorder that causes progressive degeneration of nerve cells in the brain due the aggregation of the mutant Huntingtin protein [186–188]. Lee et al. [186] investigated the therapeutic role of exosomes from adipose-derived stem cells by examining pathological phenotypes of a HD model *in vitro*. They confirmed that adipose stem cell-derived exosomes up-regulates the peroxisome proliferator-activated receptor gamma coactivator 1, phosphorylated cyclic AMP response element binding protein, and ameliorates abnormal apoptotic protein level in an *in vitro* HD model [186]. A year later, Soon-Tae Lee and colleagues developed an therapeutic exosome-based delivery method to treat HD using miR-124, one of the key miRNAs that is repressed in HD [189].

8. Exosomes in infectious diseases

8.1. Viruses

Exosomes derived from virus-infected cells have been shown to carry viral proteins, genetic regulatory elements, genomic RNA, mRNA, and miRNA [50, 190, 191]. Depending on the genetic material and proteins incorporated into them, EVs may play a vital role in viral infection, especially in retroviruses [192]. Retroviruses are enveloped RNA viruses that replicate through a DNA intermediate inserted in the host cell genome [193]. According to the Trojan hypothesis, it is believed that retroviruses exploit preexisting pathways for intracellular trafficking [192, 194]. Thus, the Trojan hypothesis states that retroviruses use the preexisting, nonviral exosome biogenesis pathway for the formation of infectious particles, and the preexisting, nonviral pathway of exosome uptake for a receptor-independent, enveloped-independent mode of infection [81, 194–196].

Among the retroviruses, HIV-1 is the most common studied virus [127, 197]. Exosomes isolated from patients with HIV infection or from HIV-1 infected cells incorporate the viral trans-activating response element that is transcribed from the integrated provirus [50, 198]. This is believed to stimulate HIV-1 replication in recipient cells by downregulation of apoptosis [50, 197–199]. Madison et al. [200] showed that semen-derived exosomes inhibit HIV-1 replication in various cell types. Years later, Madison and colleagues described detailed protocols for evaluating the function and physical properties of these semen-derived exosomes [200] for *in vitro* uptake and HIV-1 infection assays [201]. Recently, Sims et al. [92] have demonstrated the role of T cell immunoglobulin and mucin proteins (TIM) in exosome-dependent HIV-1 trafficking into human immune cells. Through viral infection assays, they demonstrated that exosomes derived from human lung carcinoma, human breast milk, human plasma, and mouse neural stem cells, increased HIV-1 entry into macrophages and T cells [92]. Furthermore, they demonstrated that HIV-1 and exosome interactions were potentially mediated through binding of TIM4 to the viral envelope [92]. In another study, Sims and colleagues demonstrated that exosomes can enhance HIV-1 entry into human monocytic and T cell lines through exosomal tetraspanin proteins CD9 and CD81 [127].

8.2. Bacteria-derived exosomes

Bacteria make and release membranous vesicles [202–204]. Gram-negative bacteria produce outer-membrane vesicles that originate from the blebbing of the outer membrane [202]. Also, they form vesicles that contain membrane components, nucleic acids, and proteins [202]. Many gram-negative bacteria that produce these vesicles are pathogenic and toxic to host cells [202, 205–207]. However, they can deliver antigens; and therefore, act as a potential vaccine candidate [202, 206, 207].

Gram-positive bacteria produce outer-membrane vesicles [202, 208]. Unlike gram-negative bacteria, these vesicles play a role in inter-species and intra-species communications [202, 209], in addition to potential inter-kingdom interaction with the host [202, 206, 210]. Most importantly, these vesicles provide an innovative approach for development of non-live vaccines [202]. These vaccines have been successfully used with children infected with *Neisseria meningitidis* in New Zealand [211].

8.3. Parasitic-derived exosomes

There is accumulating evidence that has reported the release of EVs in parasitic diseases, acting in parasite–parasite inter-communication and in parasite-host interactions [212–214]. EVs participate in the dissemination of the pathogen and play a vital role in host-pathogen interactions [212, 215]. Vesicles that are secreted by infected cells contain large amounts of pathogen molecules, which are sufficient to induce modifications in non-infected neighboring cells or act as antigen presenters for the immune system [215]. In 2013, Hassani and Olivier identified GP63 surface protease of *Leishmania mexicana* on exosomes [202, 216]. They observed that this protease could be transmitted to distant sites by enzymatic activity [202, 216].

9. Exosomes as diagnostic and therapeutic biomarkers

Exosomes have attracted enormous research interest because of their promising medical applications [217–219]. Exosomes may serve as diagnostic tools because they are carriers of molecular markers of many diseases and as a prospective delivery system for various therapeutic agents [75, 220–222]. Supporting evidence suggests that exosomes are present in all bodily fluids and may be associated with disease pathogenesis [223–226] and may be involved in cellular protection [227, 228]. Mostly importantly, they contain various nucleic acids, lipids, and proteins. Due to the cargo of exosomes, exosomes are involved in several infectious diseases [75]. Because of their endocytic origin, exosomes carry specialized protein markers, such as hsps, tetraspanin, and Rab family proteins. Exosomal content is a fingerprint of the state (cancer versus quiescent) of the cell and the original cell type.

Exosomes can be used to diagnosis various diseases, such as cancer, AD, PD, HD, etc. [150, 173, 174, 186, 229]. Non-invasive diagnostics (using saliva and urine samples) or minimum invasive diagnostics (based on blood analysis) make exosomes very attractive alternatives to excision biopsies or traditional needle biopsies. There are advantages such as lower cost analysis, convenience and reduction in patient pain [229].

Exosomes can be exploited as potential carriers for therapeutics [230]. Many anti-inflammatory drugs (i.e. Doxorubicin) can be inserted into purified exosomes for *in vivo* and *in vitro* applications [231–235]. Sun et al. [236] investigated the anti-inflammatory activities of curcumin when encapsulated in exosomes. A year later, Zhuang and colleagues demonstrated that exosomes can be utilized to deliver anti-inflammatory drugs to the brain through a non-invasive intranasal route [232].

10. Summary

Secreted exosomes have important functions in the pathogenesis of various diseases. Several methods have been developed to isolate, purify, and characterize exosomes from biological fluids. However, isolation of exosomes can be problematic during the purification process due contaminants, such as protein aggregates, microvesicles, microbes, etc. Because of theses contaminates, it is challenging to characterize exosomes accurately, and use them for experimental assays. Centrifugation techniques remain very common. However, other methods, such as filtration, sucrose density gradient centrifugation, SEC, microfluidics, and ExoQuick™ show promising results and can be effectively applied both in laboratory research and clinical medicine. It is most important to note that subsequent to exosome purification it is necessary to employ a combination of methods to confirm and characterize extracellular vesicles. The utilization of multimodality validations will allow researchers to obtain data that is qualitative, quantitative or both. Characterization of exosomes allows researchers to understand exosomal properties and function. Most importantly, characterization studies allow researchers to identify unique exosomal marker proteins to detect the presence of exosomes found in cell culture supernatants and biological fluids. The study of EV composition has shown that they can carry numerous cargos (i.e. lipids, proteins, and nucleic acids). These cargos can vary widely between cells and conditions. Their composition is cell type-dependent that can be altered by different environmental factors. The use of exosomes as therapeutic delivery vehicles covers a wide array of diseases, including but not limited to cancer, virus-induced diseases, genetically related diseases and parasitic diseases.

Acknowledgements

This work was supported by NIH/NIDA-1R15 DA045564-01 (Matthews).

Author details

Brennetta J. Crenshaw[1], Brian Sims[2] and Qiana L. Matthews[1]*

*Address all correspondence to: qmatthews@alasu.edu

1 Microbiology Program, Department of Biological Sciences, College of Science, Technology, Engineering and Mathematics, Alabama State University, AL, USA

2 Departments of Pediatrics and Cell, Developmental and Integrative Biology, Division of Neonatology, University of Alabama at Birmingham, AL, USA

References

[1] Kowal J, Tkach M, Théry C. Biogenesis and secretion of exosomes. Current Opinion in Cell Biology. 2014;**29**:116-125

[2] Brintonn LT, Sloane H, Kester M, Kelly KA. Formation and role of exosomes in cancer. Cellular and Molecular Life Sciences. 2015;**72**(4):659-671

[3] Harding C, Stahl P. Transferrin recycling in reticulocytes: pH and iron are important determinants of ligand binding and processing. Biochemical and Biophysical Research Communications. 1983;**11**(2):650-658

[4] Pan BT, Johnstone RM. Fate of the transferrin receptor during maturation of sheep reticulocytes in vitro: Selective externalization of the receptor. Cell. 1983;**33**(3):967-78

[5] De Broe ME, Wieme R, Logghe GN, Roels F. Spontaneous shedding of plasma membrane fragments by human cells in vivo and in vitro. Clinica Chimica Acta. 1977;**81**(3):237-245

[6] De Broe ME, Borgers M, Wieme RJ. The separation and characterization of liver plasma membrane fragments circulating in the blood of patients with cholestasis. Clinica Chimica Acta. 1975;**59**(3):369-372

[7] Brocklehurst D, Wilde C, Doar JW. The incidence and likely origins of serum particulate alkaline phosphatase and lipoprotein-X in liver disease. Clinica Chimica Acta. 1978; **88**(3):509-515

[8] Pan BT, Teng K, Wu C, Adam M, Johnstone RM. Electron microscopic evidence for externalization of the transferin receptor in vesicular form in sheep reticulocytes. The Journal of Cell Biology. 1985;**101**(3):942-948

[9] Johnstone RM, Adam M, Hammond JR, Orr L, Turbide C. Vesicle formation during reticulocyte maturation. Association of plasma membrane activities with released vesicles (exosomes). The Journal of Biological Chemistry. 1987;**262**(19):9412-9420

[10] Joao AM, Alenquer M. Exosome biogenesis, regulation, and function in viral infection. Viruses. 2015;**7**(9):5066-5083

[11] Harding CV, Heuser J, Stahl PD. Exosomes: Looking back three decades and into the future. The Journal of Cell Biology. 2013;**200**(4):367-371

[12] Peter W. The nature and significance of platelet products in human plasma. British Journal of Haematology. 1967;**13**(3):269-288

[13] Arraud N et al. Extracellular vesicles from blood plasma: Determination of their morphology, size, phenotype, and concentration. Journal of Thrombosis and Haemostasis. 2014;**12**(5):614-627

[14] He C, Zheng S, Luo Y, Wang B. Exosome theranostics: Biology and translational medicine. Theranostics. 2018;**8**(1):237-255

[15] Bobrie A, Colombo M, Raposo G, Théry C. Exosome secretion: Molecular mechanisms and roles in immune responses. Traffic. 2011;**12**(12):1659-1668

[16] Raposo G, Stoorvogel W. Extracellular vesicles: Exosomes, microvesicles, and friends. The Journal of Cell Biology. 2013;**200**(4):373-383

[17] Colombo M, Moita C, van Niel G, Kowal J, Vigneron J, Benaroch P, Manel N, Moita LF, Théry C, Raposo G. Analysis of ESCRT functions in exosome biogenesis, composition and secretion highlights the heterogeneity of extracellular vesicles. Journal of Cell Science. 2013;**126**(24):5553-5565

[18] Raiborg C, Stenmark H. The ESCRT machinery in endosomal sorting of ubiquitylated membrane proteins. Nature. 2009;**458**(7237):445-452

[19] Wollert T et al. The ESCRT machinery at a glance. Journal of Cell Science. 2009;**122**(13): 2163-2166

[20] Pocognoni CA, Berberián MV, Mayorga LS. ESCRT (Endosomal Sorting Complex Required for Transport) machinery is essential for acrosomal exocytosis in human sperm 1. Biology of Reproduction. 2015;**93**(5):124, 1-12-124, 1-12

[21] Christ L et al. Cellular functions and molecular mechanisms of the ESCRT membrane-scission machinery. Trends in Biochemical Sciences. 2017;**42**(1):42-56

[22] Kojima K, Amano Y, Yoshino K, Tanaka N, Sugamura K, Takeshita T. ESCRT-0 protein hepatocyte growth factor-regulated tyrosine kinase substrate (Hrs) is targeted to endosomes independently of signal-transducing adaptor molecule (STAM) and the complex formation with STAM promotes its endosomal dissociation. Journal of Biological Chemistry. 2015;**290**(13):8065-8066

[23] Meister M, Bänfer S, Gärtner U, Koskimies J, Amaddii M, Jacob R, Tikkanen R. Regulation of cargo transfer between ESCRT-0 and ESCRT-I complexes by flotillin-1 during endosomal sorting of ubiquitinated cargo. Oncogene. 2017;**6**(6):e344

[24] Wollert T et al. Membrane scission by the ESCRT-III complex. Nature. 2009;**458**:172-177

[25] Saksena S et al. ESCRTing proteins in the endocytic pathway. Trends in Biochemical Sciences. 2007;**32**(12):561-573

[26] Villarroya-Beltri C et al. Sorting it out: Regulation of exosome loading. Seminars in Cancer Biology. 2014;**28**:3-13

[27] Landsberg MJ et al. Three-dimensional structure of AAA ATPase Vps4: Advancing structural insights into the mechanisms of endosomal sorting and enveloped virus budding. Structure. 2009;**17**(3):427-437

[28] Allison B, Zhang H, Ratajczak MZ, Kakar SS. Exosomes: An overview of biogenesis, composition and role in ovarian cancer. Journal of Ovarian Research. 2014;**7**(14):1-11

[29] Henderson MC, Azorsa DO. The genomic and proteomic content of cancer cell-derived exosomes. Frontiers in Oncology. 2012;**2**(38):1-9

[30] Taylor DD, Gercel-Taylor C. Micro RNA signatures of tumor-derived exosomes as diagnostic biomarkers of ovarian cancer. Gynecologic Oncology. 2008;**110**(1):13-21

[31] Hu G, Drescher KM, Chen XM. Exosomal miRNAs: Biological properties and therapeutic potential. Frontiers in Genetics. 2012;**3**(56):1-9

[32] Chivet M, Hemming F, Pernet-Gallay K, Fraboulet S, Sadoul R. Emerging role of neuronal exosomes in the central nervous system. Frontiers in Physiology. 2012;**3**(145):1-6

[33] Van Niel G, Mallegol J, Bevilacqua C, Candalh C, Brugière S, Tomaskovic-Crook E, Heath JK, Cerf-Bensussan N, Heyman M. Intestinal epithelial exosomes carry MHC class II/peptides able to inform the immune system in mice. Gut. 2003;**52**(12):1690-1697

[34] Kapsogeorgou EK, Abu-Helu R, Moutsopoulos HM, Manoussakis MN. Salivary gland epithelial cell exosomes: A source of autoantigenic ribonucleoproteins. Arthritis and Rheumatism. 2005;**52**(5):1517-1521

[35] Théry C, Regnault A, Garin J, Wolfers J, Zitvogel L, Ricciardi-Castagnoli P, Raposo G, Amigorena S. Molecular characterization of dendritic cell-derived exosomes. Selective accumulation of the heat shock protein hsc73. The Journal of Cell Biology. 1999;**147**(3): 599-610

[36] Zech D, Rana S, Büchler MW, Zöller M. Tumor-exosomes and leukocyte activation: An ambivalent crosstalk. Cell Communication and Signaling. 2012;**10**(1):1-17

[37] Wang G, Dinkins M, He Q, Zhu G, Poirier C, Campbell A, Mayer-Proschel M, Bieberich E. Astrocytes secrete exosomes enriched with proapoptotic ceramide and prostate apoptosis response 4 (PAR-4): Potential mechanism of apoptosis induction in Alzheimer disease (AD). The Journal of Biological Chemistry. 2012;**287**(25):21384-21395

[38] Zhan R, Leng X, Liu X, Wang X, Gong J, Yan L, Wang L, Wang Y, Wang X, Qian LJ. Heat shock protein 70 is secreted from endothelial cells by a non-classical pathway involving exosomes. Biochemical and Biophysical Research Communications. 2009;**387**(2):229-233

[39] Laulagnier K, Motta C, Hamdi S, Roy S, Fauvelle F, Pageaux JF, Kobayashi T, Salles JP, Perret B, Bonnerot C, Record M. Mast cell- and dendritic cell-derived exosomes display a specific lipid composition and an unusual membrane organization. The Biochemical Journal. 2004;**380**:161-171

[40] Lai RC, Arslan F, Lee MM, Sze NS, Choo A, Chen TS, Salto-Tellez M, Timmers L, Lee CN, El Oakley RM, Pasterkamp G, de Kleijn DP, Lim SK. Exosome secreted by MSC reduces myocardial ischemia/reperfusion injury. Stem Cell Research. 2010;**4**(3):214-122

[41] Lässer C, ONS, Ekerljung L, Ekström K, Sjöstrand M, Lötvall J. RNA-containing exosomes in human nasal secretions. American Journal of Rhinology & Allergy. 2011;**25**(2):89-93

[42] Baranyai T, Herczeg K, Onódi Z, Voszka I, Módos K, Marton N, Nagy G, Mäger I, Wood MJ, El Andaloussi S, Pálinkás Z, Kumar V, Nagy P, Kittel Á, Buzás EI, Ferdinandy P, Giricz Z. Isolation of exosomes from blood plasma: Qualitative and quantitative comparison of ultracentrifugation and size exclusion chromatography methods. PLoS One. 2015;**10**(12):1-13

[43] Gallo A, Tandon M, Alevizos I, Illei GG. The majority of microRNAs detectable in serum and saliva is concentrated in exosomes. PLoS One. 2012;**7**(3):1-5

[44] Keller S, Ridinger J, Rupp AK, Janssen JW, Altevogt P. Body fluid derived exosomes as a novel template for clinical diagnostics. Journal of Translational Medicine. 2011;**9**(86):1-9

[45] Keller S, Rupp C, Stoeck A, Runz S, Fogel M, Lugert S, Hager HD, Abdel-Bakky MS, Gutwein P, Altevogt P. CD24 is a marker of exosomes secreted into urine and amniotic fluid. Kidney International. 2007;**72**(9):1095-1102

[46] Qin W, Tsukasaki Y, Dasgupta S, Mukhopadhyay N, Ikebe M, Sauter ER. Exosomes in human breast milk promote EMT. Clinical Cancer Research. 2016;**22**(17):4517-4524

[47] Record M, Subra C, Silvente-Poirot S, Poirot M. Exosomes as intercellular signalosomes and pharmacological effectors. Biochemical Pharmacology. 2011;**81**(10):1171-1182

[48] Record M. Exosomal lipids in cell-cell communication. In: Z HG, editor. Emerging Concepts of Tumor Exosome-Mediated Cell-Cell Communication. New York, NY: Springer; 2013

[49] Théry C, Ostrowski M, Segura E. Membrane vesicles as conveyors of immune responses. Nature Reviews. Immunology. 2009;**9**(8):581-593

[50] Chahar HS, Bao X, Casola A. Exosomes and their role in the life cycle and pathogenesis of RNA viruses. Viruses. 2015;**7**(3):3204-3225

[51] Record M, Carayon K, Poirot M, Silvente-Poirot S. Exosomes as new vesicular lipid transporters involved in cell-cell communication and various pathophysiologies. Biochimica et Biophysica Acta. 2014;**1841**(1):108-120

[52] Sluijter JP, Verhage V, Deddens JC, van den Akker F, Doevendans PA. Microvesicles and exosomes for intracardiac communication. Cardiovascular Research. 2014;**102**(2):302-311

[53] Ostrowski M, Carmo N, Krumeich S, Fanget I, Raposo G, Savina A, Moita CF, Schauer K, Hume AN, Freitas RP, Goud B, Benaroch P, Hacohen N, Fukuda M, Desnos C, Seabra

MC, Darchen F, Amigorena S, Moita LF, Thery C. Rab27a and Rab27b control different steps of the exosome secretion pathway. Nature Cell Biology. 2010;**12**(1):19-30

[54] Ponnambalam S, Baldwin S. Constitutive protein secretion from the trans-Golgi network to the plasma membrane (Review). 2003;**20**:129-139

[55] Stenmark H, Stenmark H. Rab GTPases as coordinators of vesicle traffic. Nature Reviews. Molecular Cell Biology. 2009;**10**:513-525

[56] Blanc L, Vidal M. New insights into the function of Rab GTPases in the context of exosomal secretion. Small GTPases. 2016;**9**(1-2):95-106

[57] Pfeffer S. Rab GTPases: Specifying and deciphering organelle identity and function. Trends in Cell Biology. 2002;**11**:487-491

[58] Hsu C, Morohashi Y, Yoshimura S, Manrique-Hoyos N, Jung SY, Lauterbach MA, Bakhti M, Grønborg M, Möbius W, Rhee JS, Barr FA, Simons M. Regulation of exosome secretion by Rab35 and its GTPase-activating proteins TBC1D10A–C. Journal of Cell Biology. 2010;**189**(2):223-232

[59] Li G, Marlin MC, Rab GTPases. In: LG, editor. Methods in Molecular Biology. New York, NY: Humana Press; 2015

[60] Hsu C, Morohashi Y, Yoshimura S, Manrique-Hoyos N, Jung S, Lauterbach MA, Bakhti M, Grønborg M, Möbius W, Rhee J, Barr FA, Simons M. Regulation of exosome secretion by Rab35 and its GTPase-activating proteins TBC1D10A. The Journal of Cell Biology. 2010;**189**(2):223-232

[61] Hessvik NP, Llorente A. Current knowledge on exosome biogenesis and release. Cellular and Molecular Life Sciences. 2018;**75**(2):193-208

[62] Savina A, Vidal M, Colombo MI. The exosome pathway in K562 cells is regulated by Rab11. Journal of Cell Science. 2002;**115**(12):2505-2515

[63] Lindsay AJ, McCaffrey MW. Rabs of the Endosomal Recycling Pathway, in Encyclopedia of Cell Biology. Waltham: Academic Press; 2016. pp. 401-407

[64] Lindsay AJ, MM. Rab11-FIP2 functions in transferrin recycling and associates with endosomal membranes via its COOH-terminal domain. The Journal of Biological Chemistry. 2002;**277**(30):27193-27199

[65] Bouchet J et al. Rab11-FIP3 regulation of lck endosomal traffic controls TCR signal transduction. The Journal of Immunology. 2017;**198**(7):2967-2978

[66] Ailawadi S, Wang X, Gu H, Fan GC. Pathologic function and therapeutic potential of exosomes in cardiovascular disease. Biochimica et Biophysica Acta. 2015;**1852**(1):1-11

[67] Yu X, Harris S, Levine AJ. The regulation of exosome secretion: A novel function of the p53 protein. Cancer Research. 2006;**66**(9):4795-4801

[68] Keller S, Sanderson M, Stoeck A, Altevogt P, Exosomes: From biogenesis and secretion to biological function. Immunology Letters. 2006;**107**(2):102-108

[69] Gross JC et al. Active Wnt proteins are secreted on exosomes. Nature Cell Biology. 2012;**14**:1036

[70] Lespagnol A, Duflaut D, Beekman C, Blanc L, Fiucci G, Marine JC, Vidal M, Amson R, Telerman A. Exosome secretion, including the DNA damage-induced p53-dependent secretory pathway, is severely compromised in TSAP6/Steap3-null mice. Cell Death and Differentiation. 2008;**15**(11):1723-1733

[71] King HW, Michael M, Gleadle JM. Hypoxic enhancement of exosome release by breast cancer cells. BMC Cancer. 2012;**212**(421):1-10

[72] Harris AL. Hypoxia—A key regulatory factor in tumour growth. Nature Reviews. Cancer. 2002;**2**(1):38-47

[73] Hooper C et al. Wnt3a induces exosome secretion from primary cultured rat microglia. 2012;**13**:144

[74] Boriachek K et al. Biological functions and current advances in isolation and detection strategies for exosome nanovesicles. Small Journal. 2017;**14**:1702153

[75] Lin J et al. Exosomes: Novel biomarkers for clinical diagnosis. The Scientific World Journal. 2015;**2015**:8

[76] Alipoor SD, Mortaz E, Garssen J, Movassaghi M, Mirsaeidi M, Adcock IM. Exosomes and exosomal miRNA in respiratory diseases. Mediators of Inflammation. 2016;**2016**:1-11

[77] Mathivanan S et al. ExoCarta 2012: Database of exosomal proteins, RNA and lipids. Nucleic Acids Research. 2012;**40**:D1241-D1244

[78] Clotilde T, Zitvogel L, Amigorena S. Exosomes: Composition, biogenesis and function. Nature Reviews Immunology. 2002;**2**:569-579

[79] Yakimchuk K. Exosomes: Isolation and characterization methods and specific markers. Labome. Mater Methods. 2015;**5**(1450):ref79retrieved from https://labome.com/method

[80] Kalluri R. The biology and function of exosomes in cancer. The Journal of Clinical Investigation. 2016;**126**(4):1208-1215

[81] Booth AM et al. Exosomes and HIV Gag bud from endosome-like domains of the T cell plasma membrane. The Journal of Cell Biology. 2006;**172**(6):923-935

[82] Bang C, Thum T. Exosomes: New players in cell–cell communication. The International Journal of Biochemistry & Cell Biology. 2012;**44**(11):2060-2064

[83] Teresa J et al. Mechanisms of RNA loading into exosomes. FEBS Letters. 2015;**589**(13): 1391-1398

[84] Zhang J et al. Exosome and exosomal microRNA: Trafficking, sorting, and function. Genomics, Proteomics & Bioinformatics. 2015;**13**(1):17-24

[85] Behbahani GD et al. The role of exosomes contents on genetic and epigenetic alterations of recipient cancer cells. Iranian Journal of Basic Medical Sciences. 2016;**19**(10):1031-1039

[86] Valadi H et al. Exosome-mediated transfer of mRNAs and microRNAs is a novel mechanism of genetic exchange between cells. Nature Cell Biology. 2007;**9**:654

[87] Szatanek R, Baran J, Siedlar M, Baj-Krzyworzeka M. Isolation of extracellular vesicles: Determining the correct approach (Review). International Journal of Molecular Medicine. 2015;**36**(1):11-17

[88] Li P, Kaslan M, Lee SH, Yao J, Gao Z. Progress in Exosome Isolation Techniques. Theranostics. 2017;**7**(3):789-804

[89] Khatun Z, Bhat A, Sharma S, Sharma A. Elucidating diversity of exosomes: Biophysical and molecular characterization methods. Nanomedicine. 2016;**11**(17):2359-2377

[90] Willis GR, Kourembanas S, Mitsialis SA. Toward exosome-based therapeutics: Isolation, heterogeneity, and fit-for-purpose potency. Frontiers in Cardiovascular Medicine. 2017; **4**(63):1-13

[91] Momen-Heravi F, Balaj L, Alian S, Mantel PY, Halleck AE, Trachtenberg AJ, Soria CE, Oquin S, Bonebreak CM, Saracoglu E, Skog J, Kuo WP, Current methods for the isolation of extracellular vesicles. Biological Chemistry. 2013;**394**(10):1253-1262

[92] Sims B, Farrow AL, Williams SD, Bansal A, Krendelchtchikov A, Gu L, Matthews QL. Role of TIM-4 in exosome-dependent entry of HIV-1 into human immune cells. International Journal of Nanomedicine. 2017;**12**:4823-4833

[93] Sims B, Gu L, Krendelchtchikov A, Matthews QL. Neural stem cell-derived exosomes mediate viral entry. International Journal of Nanomedicine. 2014;**9**:4893-4897

[94] Nordin J, Lee Y, Vader P, Mäger I, Johansson HJ, Heusermann W, Wiklander OP, Hällbrink M, Seow Y, Bultema JJ, Gilthorpe J, Davies T1, Fairchild PJ, Gabrielsson S, Meisner Kober NC, Lehtiö J, Smith CI, Wood MJ, El Andaloussi S. Ultrafiltration with size-exclusion liquid chromatography for high yield isolation of extracellular vesicles preserving intact biophysical and functional properties. Nanomedicine. 2015;**11**(4):879-883

[95] Théry C et al. Isolation and characterization of exosomes from cell culture supernatants and biological fluids. Current Protocols in Cell Biology. 2006;**30**(1):3.22.1-3.22.29

[96] Raposo G, Nijman HW, Stoorvogel W, Liejendekker R, Harding CV, Melief CJ, Geuze HJ. B lymphocytes secrete antigen-presenting vesicles. The Journal of Experimental Medicine. 1996;**183**(3):1161-1172

[97] Cantin R, Diou J, Bélanger D, Tremblay AM, Gilbert C. Discrimination between exosomes and HIV-1: Purification of both vesicles from cell-free supernatants. Journal of Immunological Methods. 2008;**338**(1-2):21-30

[98] Lozano-Ramos I, Bancu I, Oliveira-Tercero A, et al. Size-exclusion chromatography-based enrichment of extracellular vesicles from urine samples. Journal of Extracellular Vesicles. 2015;**4**:1-11

[99] Taylor DD, LK, Gerçel-Taylor C. Shed membrane fragment-associated markers for endometrial and ovarian cancers. Gynecologic Oncology. 2002;**84**(3):443-448

[100] Feng Y, Huang W, Wani M, Yu X, Ashraf M. Ischemic preconditioning potentiates the protective effect of stem cells through secretion of exosomes by targeting Mecp2 via miR-22. PLOS One. 2014;**9**(2):1-8

[101] Rood IM, DJ, Merchant ML, Tamboer WP, Wilkey DW, Wetzels JF, et al, Comparison of three methods for isolation of urinary microvesiclesto identify biomarkers of nephrotic syndrome. Kidney International. 2010;**78**:810-816

[102] Musante L, Tataruch DE, Holthofer H, Use and isolation of urinary exosomes as biomarkers for diabetic nephropathy. Frontiers in Endocrinology. 2014;**5**(149).1-12

[103] Velve-Casquillas G, Le Berre M, Piel M, Tran PT. Microfluidic tools for cell biological research. Nano Today. 2010;**5**(1):28-47

[104] Huang-Doran I, Zhang C-Y, Vidal-Puig A. Extracellular vesicles: Novel mediators of cell communication in metabolic disease. Trends in Endocrinology & Metabolism. 2017;**28**(1):3-18

[105] Gholizadeh S et al. Microfluidic approaches for isolation, detection, and characterization of extracellular vesicles: Current status and future directions. Biosensors and Bioelectronics. 2017;**91**:588-605

[106] Halldorsson S et al. Advantages and challenges of microfluidic cell culture in polydimethylsiloxane devices. Biosensors and Bioelectronics. 2015;**63**:218-231

[107] Streets AM, Huang Y. Chip in a lab: Microfluidics for next generation life science research. Biomicrofluidics. 2013;**7**(1):011302

[108] Caradec J et al. Reproducibility and efficiency of serum-derived exosome. Extraction methods. Clinical Biochemistry. 2014;**47**:1286-1292

[109] Rider MA, Hurwitz SN, Meckes D. ExtraPEG: A polyethylene glycol-based method for enrichment of extracellular vesicles. Scientific Reports. 2016;**6**:23978

[110] Kenigsberg S et al. Protocol for exosome isolation from small volume of ovarian follicular fluid: Evaluation of ultracentrifugation and commercial kits. In: Kuo WP, Jia S, editors. Extracellular Vesicles: Methods and Protocols. New York, NY: Springer; 2017. pp. 321-341

[111] System Biosciences. ExoQuick. Retrieved from https://www.systembio.com/

[112] Barreiro K, Holthofer H. Urinary extracellular vesicles. A promising shortcut to novel biomarker discoveries. Cell and Tissue Research. 2017;**369**(1):217-227

[113] Verma M et al. Extracellular vesicles: Potential applications in cancer diagnosis, prognosis, and epidemiology. BMC Clinical Pathology. 2015;**15**(1):6

[114] Yamada T, Inoshima Y, Matsuda T, Ishiguro N. Comparison of methods for isolating exosomes from bovine milk. The Journal of Veterinary Medical Science. 2012;**74**(11): 1523-1525

[115] Shin H et al. High-yield isolation of extracellular vesicles using aqueous two-phase system. Scientific Reports. 2015;**5**:13103

[116] Kim HK et al. Optimized flow cytometric assay for the measurement of platelet microparticles in plasma: Pre-analytic and analytic considerations. Blood Coagulation & Fibrinolysis. 2002;**13**(5):393-397

[117] Szatanek R et al. The methods of choice for extracellular vesicles (EVs) characterization. International Journal of Molecular Sciences. 2017;**18**(6):1-18

[118] Mehdiani A et al. An innovative method for exosome quantification and size measurement. Journal of Visualized Experiments. 2015;**95**(e50974):1-9

[119] Tirinato L et al. SERS analysis on exosomes using super-hydrophobic surfaces. Microelectronic Engineering. 2012;**97**:337-340

[120] Lasser C, Eldh M, Lotvall J. Isolation and characterization of RNA-containing exosomes. Journal of Visualized Experiments. 2012;**59**:e3037

[121] Momen-Heravi F et al. Alternative methods for characterization of extracellular vesicles. Frontiers in Physiology. 2012;**3**:354

[122] van der Pol E et al. Single vs. swarm detection of microparticles and exosomes by flow cytometry. Journal of Thrombosis and Haemostasis. 2012;**10**(5):919-930

[123] Welsh JA et al. Extracellular vesicle flow cytometry analysis and standardization. Frontiers in Cell and Development Biology. 2017;**5**:78

[124] Morales-Kastresana A, Jones JC. Flow cytometric analysis of extracellular vesicles. Methods in Molecular Biology. 2017;**1545**:215-225

[125] Witwer KW et al. Standardization of sample collection, isolation and analysis methods in extracellular vesicle research. Journal of Extracellular Vesicles. 2013;**2**:1-25

[126] Dragovic RA et al. Sizing and phenotyping of cellular vesicles using nanoparticle tracking analysis. Nanomedicine. 2011;**7**(6):780-788

[127] Sims B et al. Tetraspanin blockage reduces exosome-mediated HIV-1 entry. Archives of Virology. 2018;**163**(6):1683-1689

[128] Filipe V, Hawe A, Jiskoot W. Critical evaluation of nanoparticle tracking analysis (NTA) by NanoSight for the measurement of nanoparticles and protein aggregates. Pharmaceutical Research. 2010;**27**(5):796-810

[129] Smith ZJ et al. Single exosome study reveals subpopulations distributed among cell lines with variability related to membrane content. Journal of Extracellular Vesicles. 2015;**4**:28533

[130] Puppels GJ et al. Studying single living cells and chromosomes by confocal Raman microspectroscopy. Nature. 1990;**347**(6290):301-303

[131] van der Pol E et al. Optical and non-optical methods for detection and characterization of microparticles and exosomes. Journal of Thrombosis and Haemostasis. 2010; **8**(12):2596-2607

[132] Tatischeff I et al. Fast characterisation of cell-derived extracellular vesicles by nanoparticles tracking analysis, cryo-electron microscopy, and Raman tweezers microspectroscopy. Journal of Extracellular Vesicles. 2012;**1**:1-11

[133] Sunkara V, Woo HK, Cho YK. Emerging techniques in the isolation and characterization of extracellular vesicles and their roles in cancer diagnostics and prognostics. Analyst. 2016;**141**(2):371-381

[134] Rho J et al. Magnetic nanosensor for detection and profiling of erythrocyte-derived microvesicles. ACS Nano. 2013;**7**(12):11227-11233

[135] He M et al. Integrated immunoisolation and protein analysis of circulating exosomes using microfluidic technology. Lab on a Chip. 2014;**14**(19):3773-3780

[136] Simpson RJ, Kalra H, Mathivanan S. ExoCarta as a resource for exosomal research. Journal of Extracellular Vesicles. 2012;**1**:1-6

[137] Wubbolts R et al. Proteomic and biochemical analyses of human B cell-derived exosomes. Potential implications for their function and multivesicular body formation. The Journal of Biological Chemistry. 2003;**278**(13):10963-10972

[138] Abramowicz A, Widlak P, Pietrowska M. Proteomic analysis of exosomal cargo: The challenge of high purity vesicle isolation. Molecular BioSystems. 2016;**12**(5):1407-1419

[139] Sharma S et al. Quantitative nanostructural and single-molecule force spectroscopy biomolecular analysis of human-saliva-derived exosomes. Langmuir. 2011;**27**(23): 14394-14400

[140] Schachermeyer S, Ashby J, Zhong W. Advances in field-flow fractionation for the analysis of biomolecules: Instrument design and hyphenation. Analytical and Bioanalytical Chemistry. 2012;**404**(4):1151-1158

[141] Graham MD. The Coulter principle: Imaginary origins. Cytometry. Part A. 2013;**83**(12): 1057-1061

[142] Ung TH et al. Exosome proteomics reveals transcriptional regulator proteins with potential to mediate downstream pathways. Cancer Science. 2014;**105**(11):1384-1392

[143] Skog J et al. Glioblastoma microvesicles transport RNA and proteins that promote tumour growth and provide diagnostic biomarkers. Nature Cell Biology. 2008;**10**(12):1470-1476

[144] Guo W et al. Exosomes: New players in cancer (Review). Oncology Reports. 2017;**38**(2): 665-675

[145] Boelens MC et al. Exosome transfer from stromal to breast cancer cells regulates therapy resistance pathways. Cell. 2014;**159**(3):499-513

[146] Oves M et al. Exosomes: A paradigm in drug development against cancer and infectious diseases. Journal of Nanomaterials. 2018;**2018**:17

[147] Zhang X et al. Exosomes in cancer: Small particle, big player. Journal of Hematology & Oncology. 2015;**8**:83

[148] Andre Mdo R, Pedro A, Lyden D. Cancer exosomes as mediators of drug resistance. Methods in Molecular Biology. 2016;**1395**:229-239

[149] Yu DD et al. Exosomes in development, metastasis and drug resistance of breast cancer. Cancer Science. 2015;**106**(8):959-964

[150] Bach DH et al. The role of exosomes and miRNAs in drug-resistance of cancer cells. International Journal of Cancer. 2017;**141**(2):220-230

[151] Wang X et al. Exosomes play an important role in the process of psoralen reverse multidrug resistance of breast cancer. Journal of Experimental & Clinical Cancer Research. 2016;**35**(1):186

[152] Ohno S-i, Ishikawa A, Kuroda M. Roles of exosomes and microvesicles in disease pathogenesis. Advanced Drug Delivery Reviews. 2013;**65**(3):398-401

[153] Corcoran C, RS, O'Brien K, O'Neill A, Prencipe M, Sheikh R, et al. Docetaxel-resistance in prostate cancer: Evaluating associated phenotypic changes and potential for resistance transfer via exosomes. PLoS One. 2012;**7**(12):e50999

[154] Akao Y et al. Extracellular disposal of tumor-suppressor miRs-145 and -34a via microvesicles and 5-FU resistance of human colon cancer cells. International Journal of Molecular Sciences. 2014;**15**(1):1392-1401

[155] Azmi AS, Bao B, Sarkar FH. Exosomes in cancer development, metastasis, and drug resistance: A comprehensive review. Cancer Metastasis Reviews. 2013;**32**(3-4):623-642

[156] Weidle UH et al. The multiple roles of exosomes in metastasis. Cancer Genomics Proteomics. 2017;**14**(1):1-15

[157] Zhang C et al. Exosome: Function and role in cancer metastasis and drug resistance. Technology in Cancer Research & Treatment. 2018;**17**:1533033818763450

[158] Becker A et al. Extracellular vesicles in cancer: Cell-to-cell mediators of metastasis. Cancer Cell. 2016;**30**(6):836-848

[159] Grange C et al. Microvesicles released from human renal cancer stem cells stimulate angiogenesis and formation of lung premetastatic niche. Cancer Research. 2011; **71**(15):5346-5356

[160] Polet F, Feron O. Endothelial cell metabolism and tumour angiogenesis: Glucose and glutamine as essential fuels and lactate as the driving force. Journal of Internal Medicine. 2013;**273**(2):156-165

[161] Abd Elmageed ZY et al. Neoplastic reprogramming of patient-derived adipose stem cells by prostate cancer cell-associated exosomes. Stem Cells. 2014;**32**(4):983-997

[162] Kahlert C, Kalluri R. Exosomes in tumor microenvironment influence cancer progression and metastasis. Journal of Molecular Medicine (Berl). 2013;**91**(4):431-437

[163] Kalra H, D.G., Mathivanan S, Focus on extracellular vesicles: Introducing the next small big thing. International Journal of Molecular Sciences. 2016;**17**(2):1-30

[164] Logozzi M et al. High levels of exosomes expressing CD63 and caveolin-1 in plasma of melanoma patients. PLoS One. 2009;**4**(4):e5219

[165] Whiteside TL. Tumor-derived exosomes and their role in cancer progression. Advances in Clinical Chemistry. 2016;**74**:103-141

[166] Atay S, Godwin AK. Tumor-derived exosomes: A message delivery system for tumor progression. Communicative & Integrative Biology. 2014;**7**(1):e28231

[167] Kogure T et al. Intercellular nanovesicle-mediated microRNA transfer: A mechanism of environmental modulation of hepatocellular cancer cell growth. Hepatology. 2011;**54**(4):1237-1248

[168] Tan A, De La Pena H, Seifalian AM. The application of exosomes as a nanoscale cancer vaccine. International Journal of Nanomedicine. 2010;**5**:889-900

[169] Ichim TE et al. Exosomes as a tumor immune escape mechanism: Possible therapeutic implications. Journal of Translational Medicine. 2008;**6**:37

[170] Kawikova I, Askenase PW. Diagnostic and therapeutic potentials of exosomes in CNS diseases. Brain Research. 2015;**1617**:63-71

[171] Rajendran L et al. Emerging roles of extracellular vesicles in the nervous system. The Journal of Neuroscience. 2014;**34**(46):15482-15489

[172] Kanninen KM et al. Exosomes as new diagnostic tools in CNS diseases. Biochimica et Biophysica Acta. 2016;**1862**(3):403-410

[173] Xiao T et al. The role of exosomes in the pathogenesis of Alzheimer' disease. Translational Neurodegeneration. 2017;**6**:3

[174] Wu X, Zheng T, Zhang B. Exosomes in Parkinson's disease. Neuroscience Bulletin. 2017;**33**(3):331-338

[175] Vella L, Hill A, Cheng L. Focus on extracellular vesicles: Exosomes and their role in protein trafficking and biomarker potential in Alzheimer's and Parkinson's disease. International Journal of Molecular Sciences. 2016;**17**:173

[176] Yuyama K et al. A potential function for neuronal exosomes: Sequestering intracerebral amyloid-β peptide. FEBS Letters. 2014;**589**

[177] Geschwind MD. Prion diseases. Continuum (Minneap. Minn.). 2015;**21**(6 Neuroinfectious Disease):1612-1638

[178] Baksi S, Singh N. Alpha-synuclein impairs ferritinophagy in the retinal pigment epithelium: Implications for retinal iron dyshomeostasis in Parkinson's disease. Scientific Reports. 2017;**7**(1):12843

[179] Karnati HK et al. miRNAs: Key players in neurodegenerative disorders and epilepsy. Journal of Alzheimer's Disease. 2015;**48**(3):563-580

[180] Wang G et al. Variation in the miRNA-433 binding site of FGF20 confers risk for Parkinson disease by overexpression of alpha-synuclein. American Journal of Human Genetics. 2008;**82**(2):283-289

[181] Doxakis E. Post-transcriptional regulation of alpha-synuclein expression by mir-7 and mir-153. The Journal of Biological Chemistry. 2010;**285**(17):12726-12734

[182] Burchell JT, Panegyres PK. Prion diseases: Immunotargets and therapy. ImmunoTargets and Therapy. 2016;**5**:57-68

[183] Soria F et al. Exosomes, an unmasked culprit in neurodegenerative diseases. Frontiers in Neuroscience. 2017;**11**:1-12

[184] Fevrier B et al. Cells release prions in association with exosomes. Proceedings of the National Academy of Sciences of the United States of America. 2004;**101**(26):9683-9688

[185] Vella LJ et al. Enrichment of prion protein in exosomes derived from ovine cerebral spinal fluid. Veterinary Immunology and Immunopathology. 2008;**124**(3-4):385-393

[186] Lee M et al. Exosomes from adipose-derived stem cells ameliorate Huntington's disease phenotypes in an in vitro model. European Journal of Neuroscience. 2016;**44**:2114-2119

[187] Hong Y et al. Mutant Huntingtin inhibits αB-crystallin expression and impairs exosome secretion from astrocytes. The Journal of Neuroscience. 2017;**37**(39):9550-9563

[188] Sari Y. Huntington's disease: From mutant Huntingtin protein to neurotrophic factor therapy. International Journal of Biomedical Science. 2011;**7**(2):89-100

[189] Lee S-T et al. Exosome-based delivery of miR-124 in a Huntington's disease model. Journal of Movement Disorders. 2017;**10**:45-52

[190] Anderson MR, Kashanchi F, Jacobson S. Exosomes in viral disease. Neurotherapeutics. 2016;**13**(3):535-546

[191] Raab-Traub N, Dittmer DP. Viral effects on the content and function of extracellular vesicles. Nature Reviews. Microbiology. 2017;**15**(9):559-572

[192] Nolte-'t Hoen E et al. Extracellular vesicles and viruses: Are they close relatives? Proceedings of the National Academy of Sciences of the United States of America. 2016;**113**(33):9155-9161

[193] Coffin JM, Hughes SH, Varmus HE, editors. Retroviruses. Cold Spring Harbor (NY): Cold Spring Harbor Laboratory Press; 1997

[194] Gould SJ, Booth AM, Hildreth JE. The Trojan exosome hypothesis. Proceedings of the National Academy of Sciences of the United States of America. 2003;**100**(19):10592-10597

[195] Hildreth JEK. HIV as trojan exosome: Immunological paradox explained? Frontiers in Immunology. 2017;**8**:1715

[196] Nguyen DG et al. Evidence that HIV budding in primary macrophages occurs through the exosome release pathway. The Journal of Biological Chemistry. 2003;**278**(52):52347-52354

[197] Ellwanger JH, Veit TD, Chies JAB. Exosomes in HIV infection: A review and critical look. Infection, Genetics and Evolution. 2017;**53**:146-154

[198] Madison MN, Okeoma CM. Exosomes: Implications in HIV-1 pathogenesis. Viruses. 2015;**7**(7):4093-4118

[199] Narayanan A et al. Exosomes derived from HIV-1-infected cells contain trans-activation response element RNA. The Journal of Biological Chemistry. 2013;**288**(27):20014-20033

[200] Madison MN, Roller RJ, Okeoma CM. Human semen contains exosomes with potent anti-HIV-1 activity. Retrovirology. 2014;**11**:102

[201] Madison MN, Welch JL, Okeoma CM. Isolation of exosomes from semen for in vitro uptake and HIV-1 infection assays. Bio-protocol. 2017;**7**(7):1-27

[202] Schwab A et al. Extracellular vesicles from infected cells: Potential for direct pathogenesis. Frontiers in Microbiology. 2015;**6**:1132

[203] Deatherage BL, Cookson BT. Membrane vesicle release in bacteria, eukaryotes, and archaea: A conserved yet underappreciated aspect of microbial life. Infection and Immunity. 2012;**80**(6):1948-1957

[204] Rodrigues M et al. Role of extracellular vesicles in viral and bacterial infections: Pathogenesis, diagnostics, and therapeutics. Theranostics. 2018;**8**(10):2709-2721

[205] Kadurugamuwa JL, Beveridge TJ. Membrane vesicles derived from *Pseudomonas aeruginosa* and *Shigella flexneri* can be integrated into the surfaces of other gram-negative bacteria. Microbiology. 1999;**145**(Pt 8):2051-2060

[206] Pierson T et al. Proteomic characterization and functional analysis of outer membrane vesicles of *Francisella novicida* suggests possible role in virulence and use as a vaccine. Journal of Proteome Research. 2011;**10**(3):954-967

[207] Nieves W et al. A Burkholderia pseudomallei outer membrane vesicle vaccine provides protection against lethal sepsis. Clinical and Vaccine Immunology. 2014;**21**(5):747-754

[208] Brown L et al. Extracellular vesicles produced by the Gram-positive bacterium *Bacillus subtilis* are disrupted by the lipopeptide surfactin. Molecular Microbiology. 2014; **93**(1):183-198

[209] Berleman J, Auer M. The role of bacterial outer membrane vesicles for intra- and interspecies delivery. Environmental Microbiology. 2013;**15**(2):347-354

[210] Kulp A, Kuehn MJ. Biological functions and biogenesis of secreted bacterial outer membrane vesicles. Annual Review of Microbiology. 2010;**64**:163-184

[211] Wong SH et al. Immunogenicity and tolerability in infants of a New Zealand epidemic strain meningococcal B outer membrane vesicle vaccine. The Pediatric Infectious Disease Journal. 2009;**28**(5):385-390

[212] Marcilla A et al. Extracellular vesicles in parasitic diseases. Journal of Extracellular Vesicles. 2014;**3**:25040

[213] Coakley G, Maizels RM, Buck AH. Exosomes and other extracellular vesicles: The new communicators in parasite infections. Trends in Parasitology. 2015;**31**(10):477-489

[214] Pontes L et al. Biomarkers in exosomes in cattle diseases. Research Gate. 2018. Conference article

[215] Atayde VD et al. Exosome secretion by the parasitic protozoan leishmania within the sand fly midgut. Cell Reports. 2015;**13**(5):957-967

[216] Hassani K, Olivier M. Immunomodulatory impact of leishmania-induced macrophage exosomes: A comparative proteomic and functional analysis. PLoS Neglected Tropical Diseases. 2013;**7**(5):e2185

[217] Dorayappan KDP et al. The biological significance and clinical applications of exosomes in ovarian cancer. Gynecologic Oncology. 2016;**142**(1):199-205

[218] Gyorgy B et al. Therapeutic applications of extracellular vesicles: Clinical promise and open questions. Annual Review of Pharmacology and Toxicology. 2015;**55**:439-464

[219] Santangelo L et al. Functional roles and therapeutic applications of exosomes in *Hepatocellular Carcinoma*. BioMed Research International. 2017;**2017**:8

[220] De Toro J, Waldner C, Mongini C. Emerging roles of exosomes in normal and pathological conditions: New insights for diagnosis and therapeutic applications. Frontiers in Immunology. 2015;**6**(203):1-12

[221] Lasser C. Exosomes in diagnostic and therapeutic applications: Biomarker, vaccine and RNA interference delivery vehicle. Expert Opinion on Biological Therapy. 2015;**15**(1):103-117

[222] Dommelen S et al. Microvesicles and exosomes: Opportunities for cell-derived membrane vesicles in drug delivery;**161, 2011**:635-644

[223] Cappello F et al. Exosome levels in human body fluids: A tumor marker by themselves? European Journal of Pharmaceutical Sciences. 2017;**96**:93-98

[224] Barile L, Vassalli G. Exosomes: Therapy delivery tools and biomarkers of diseases. Pharmacology & Therapeutics. 2017;**174**:63-78

[225] Delenclos M et al. Investigation of endocytic pathways for the internalization of exosome-associated oligomeric alpha-synuclein. Frontiers in Neuroscience. 2017;**11**(172)

[226] Zhang W et al. Exosomes in pathogen infections: A bridge to deliver molecules and link functions. Frontiers in Immunology. 2018;**9**(90):1-12

[227] Messenger SW, Woo SS, Sun Z, Martin TFJ. A Ca(2+)-stimulated exosome release pathway in cancer cells is regulated by Munc13-4. The Journal of Cell Biology. 2018;**217**(8):2877-2890

[228] Baixauli F, López-Otín C, Mittelbrunn M. Exosomes and autophagy: Coordinated mechanisms for the maintenance of cellular fitness. Frontiers in Immunology. 2014;**5**:1-627

[229] Vlassov AV et al. Exosomes: Current knowledge of their composition, biological functions, and diagnostic and therapeutic potentials. Biochimica et Biophysica Acta. 2012;**1820**(7):940-948

[230] Kooijmans SA et al. Exosome mimetics: A novel class of drug delivery systems. International Journal of Nanomedicine. 2012;**7**:1525-1541

[231] Lai RC et al. Exosomes for drug delivery—A novel application for the mesenchymal stem cell. Biotechnology Advances. 2013;**31**(5):543-551

[232] Zhuang X et al. Treatment of brain inflammatory diseases by delivering exosome encapsulated anti-inflammatory drugs from the nasal region to the brain. Molecular Therapy. 2011;**19**(10):1769-1779

[233] Alexander M et al. Exosome-delivered microRNAs modulate the inflammatory response to endotoxin. Nature Communications. 2015;**6**:7321

[234] Gupta A, Pulliam L. Exosomes as mediators of neuroinflammation. Journal of Neuroinflammation. 2014;**11**:68

[235] Yang Y et al. Increased anti-tumour activity by exosomes derived from doxorubicin-treated tumour cells via heat stress. International Journal of Hyperthermia. 2015;**31**(5):498-506

[236] Sun D et al. A novel nanoparticle drug delivery system: The anti-inflammatory activity of curcumin is enhanced when encapsulated in exosomes. Molecular Therapy. 2010;**18**(9):1606-1614

Chapter 2

Transethosomes and Nanoethosomes: Recent Approach on Transdermal Drug Delivery System

Koushlesh Kumar Mishra, Chanchal Deep Kaur,
Shekhar Verma, Anil Kumar Sahu,
Deepak Kumar Dash, Pankaj Kashyap and
Saraswati Prasad Mishra

Additional information is available at the end of the chapter

http://dx.doi.org/10.5772/intechopen.81152

Abstract

In the past few decades, an emerging drug delivery system that came into light is transdermal drug delivery system. It has become the talk of the town in the field of drug delivery because of its better and easy accessibility. Though it is one of the attractive routes, transport of drug through the skin has remained a challenge. To overcome the challenge, vesicular system has been adopted so as to have better skin permeation of bioactive agents. Vesicular system like liposome has shown inefficiency to cross the layers of skin. Then transethosomes and nanoethosomes are employed for delivering drug into the deeper layer of skin. Nanoethosomes and transethosomes have same composition that is water, ethanol and phospholipid. Transethosome contains edge activator additionally. Due to the presence of ethanol and edge activator, it displayed enhanced skin permeation. Vesicular system gives a better patient compliance, being a non-invasive method of drug administration. In this chapter, we attempted to provide brief information about methods of preparation, characterization and pharmaceutical uses of nanoethosomes and transethosomes.

Keywords: transdermal, transethosomes, nanoethosomes

1. Introduction

In last few decades many significant advancement in the field of drug delivery technology have been made. This advancement took place as there was no remarkable growth in developing new drug entities. Drug delivery emerged as a branch of science which comprises of biopharmaceutics and pharmacokinetics. Drug delivery technology is accepted as it imparts therapeutic as well as economical values to the health care products. The above said characteristic of drug delivery technology helps the old drugs to stand the competition of growing market. Drug delivery enhances the efficacy of drugs through controlled release by considering the factors like carrier system, route of administration and target of drug action. Drug delivery system improves patient compliance, therapeutic index and bioavailability [1].

In present scenario researchers are working on delivering the active pharmaceutical ingredient through transdermal route but still the effective delivery of drug through the said route is challenging. Transdermal drug delivery system originated in the year 1950 in U.S. In transdermal system drug permeate from the outer layer of skin to the blood stream through various layers of skin [2]. Transdermal drug delivery system is advantageous over traditional method. Drug administered through transdermal drug delivery system does not pass through GI Tract so are not exposed to degradation in the gut. As transdermal system delivers drug directly into blood stream through layers of skin, so drugs bypasses pre-systemic metabolism. Transdermal system is most suitable for drugs with short half life and narrow therapeutic range. The system helps in maintaining controlled level of plasma, in case of toxicity drug administration can be easily stopped. Few disadvantages are also attached to this system, such as drugs requiring blood volume cannot be administered [3–7]. Due the patches and the adhesive used in it, few recipients may experience skin irritation. For some section of patients it may not be economical. In the process of developing transdermal drug delivery system few basic areas has to be considered such as drug's bioactivity, the characteristics of skin, formulation employed, adhesive to be used and the design of the system. Permeation of drug through skin is dependent on factors like structure of skin and properties associated with it, the physicochemical property of the penetration molecule in relationship with the skin and lastly the system that carries the drug to the skin for penetration [8–10].

For overcoming the limitation of barrier function of skin some methods are undertaken such as iontophoresis, sonophoresis, electrophoresis along with micro-invasive techniques, vesicular system and employment of permeation enhancers [11, 12]. Transdermal system of drug delivery transports bioactive agents directly into blood stream. Transdermal system has many benefits like it bypasses first pass metabolism, it ensures better patient compliance and with this system there is mere chances of any kind of tissue injury. Currently vesicular system is mostly studied approach for transdermal drug delivery system. Vesicular system contains vesicles which are composed of colloids with hydrophilic and amphiphilic groups. Hydrophilic part makes the core and it is guarded by amphiphilic part in a bilayer effusion. The vesicular system act as a carrier for drugs which may be hydrophilic, lipophilic or amphiphilic. The vesicles have the ability of encapsulating the said drug types. Factors such as size, lamellarity, thermodynamic phase, surface charge are determinant of the efficiency of vesicular system as carrier [13].

Presently various type of vesicular carrier systems are available such as liposomes, ethosomes, transferosomes, niosomes, transethosomes etc. (**Figure 1**). All of them have their particular merits and demerits. There is not a single vesicular carrier that can fulfill all the criteria of drug delivery. In this chapter we are mainly focus on transethosomes and nanoethosomes vesicular carrier system.

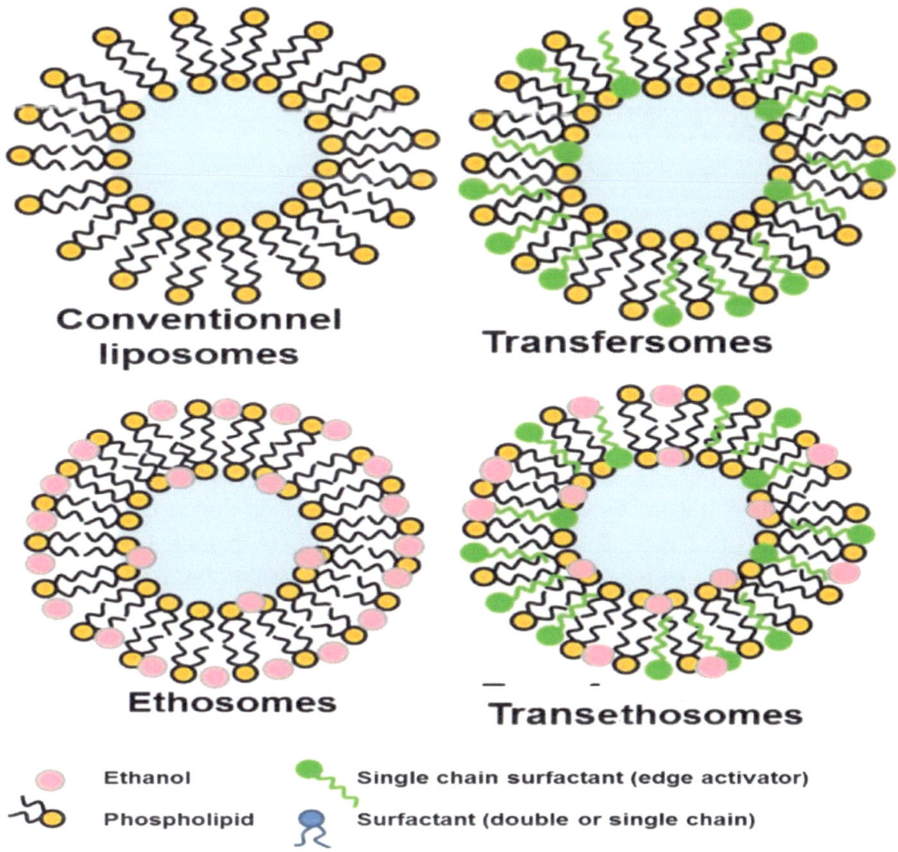

Figure 1. Schematic illustration of a panel of lipid-based nanocarrier transdermal delivery systems.

2. Transethosomes

Liposomes, which are conventional lipid-based vesicular system, are not capable of crossing the stratum corneum. As they exhibit low permeation into deeper layer of skin, eventually they get accumulated on superior layer of stratum corneum. To improve the skin permeation, liposomes are added with edge activators like Span 80, Span 25, Tween 80, sodium cholate and are named as transferosomes. Transferosomes enhances skin permeation due to their deformable ability but they are unable to penetrate deep into the stratum corneum. Another vesicular system called ethosomes is also available. Ethosomes are composed of phospholipid, ethanol and water (**Table 1**). Due to presence of ethanol the intercellular space between the corneocytes increases which increase the permeation [14–16].

Transethosomes are the combination of transferosome and ethosomes. Transferosomes shows both the quality of becoming deformable and skin permeation. This vesicular system was introduced in the year 2012 by Song et al. Transethosomes can be taken by topical as well as

S. No.	Additives	Liposomes	Ethosomes	Transethosomes	Examples	Uses
1.	Phospholipid	Present	Present	Present	Soya phosphatidyl choline	Vesicle forming component
2.	Polyglycol	Absent	Present	Present	Propylene glycol	Skin penetration enhancer
3.	Alcohol	Absent	Present	Present	Ethanol	Softness for vesicle membrane
4	Cholesterol	Present	Present	Present	cholesterol	Stability provider to vesicle membrane
5.	Vehicle	Present	Present	Present	Carbopol D934	Gel former
6.	Surfactant	Absent	Absent	Present	Sodium cholate	Edge activator

Table 1. Composition of different lipid vesicular carrier system.

systemic route. Drugs ranging from low molecular weight to high molecular weight can easily be entrapped by this system. As the bioactive agent is protected due to encapsulation, so it releases its content in a very slow and gradual manner. Due to their biodegradable and biocompatible nature, it shows highly efficient entrapment ability. Its preparation does not require any undue pharmaceutical additives and no tedious process is involved in it [15–17].

3. Nanoethosomes

Ethosomes are non-invasive carriers that assist the bioactive agents to penetrate deep into the layers of skin or into the blood stream [18]. This is a modified version of liposomal carrier system. They contains lipid vesicle along with water and ethanol. Ethosome was developed in the year 1996 by Touitou [19]. Ethosomes are known to release the entrapped bioactive agents in a constant and gradual manner. Ethosomes comes in various size. Ethosomes of nanometer size are called nanoethosomes. Presence of high content of ethanol imparts a negative charge on surface of vesicles which promotes reduction of its size [20]. Due to smaller size, nano-ethosomes easily penetrate through the intercellular space [6].

4. Advantages and disadvantages of vesicular carriers

Many vesicular formulations for drug administration through parenteral, topical as well as oral route have been developed. Vesicular drugs provides advantages like convenience, safer way of drug administration and most importantly it provides a protection for the active constituent in in-vivo condition from premature degradation. In addition to the said advantages vesicular carriers makes it possible to release encapsulated molecule in sustained and controlled manner. Due to this pattern of release it becomes easy to ensure targeted delivery of drug to the target tissues. Challenges like pre-systemic metabolism, frequent dosing, and variation in GI absorption of drug can be overcome by vesicular carriers. Vesicular carriers reduce the dosing frequency due to which the cost to the patient decreases and ensures better patient compliance. Vesicular carrier increases the bioavailability as it enhances the permeation of drug through biological carriers. Only disadvantage associated with vesicular carrier is that few patients reported symptoms of dermatitis.

4.1. Advantages and disadvantages of transethosomes

Advantages of transethosomes are that it provides semisolid dosage form for administration which gives a better patient compliance. Transethosomes ensures an enhanced permeation of drug through skin. It bypasses presystemic metabolism. Few disadvantages of transethosomes are like dermatitis, allergic reaction or skin irritation in some patients. Some product gets lost as it is transferred from alcoholic media to aqueous media [21, 22].

4.2. Advantages and disadvantages of nanoethosomes

Nanoethosomes as a carrier makes it possible to deliver large molecules like proteins. The material used to prepare nanoethosomes is non-toxic, so it is not at all harmful for the recipient. As it is easy to use, so it provides better patient compliance. As compared to methods like phonophoresis, iontophoresis it is simple method of drug delivery. Few disadvantages are also associated with nanoethosomes such as it does not provide a rapid bolus drug input. To gain entry into blood circulation the drug has to be soluble in both lipophilic and aqueous phase. Adhesives used in nanoethosomes may not adhere on the skin of every single patient. A particular molecular size of drug can be can be delivered by this system. It may not be economical for certain segment of patients [23–25].

S. No.	Carriers/method	Advantage	Disadvantage
1.	Liposomes	Phospholipid vesicle, biocompatible	Less skin penetration less stable
2.	Physical methods, e.g., iontophoresis	Increase penetration of intermediate size charged molecule	Only for charged drugs, transfer efficiency is low (less than 10%)
3.	Niosomes	Non-ionic surfactants vesicles	Less skin penetration easy handling but will not reach up to deeper skin layer
4.	Transferosomes and protransferosomes	More stable, high penetration due to high deformability, biocompatible and biodegradable, suitable for both low and high molecular weight and also for lipophilic as well as hydrophilic drugs and reach up to deeper skin layers.	None, but for some limitations
5.	Transethosomes	• Enhanced drug permeation through skin for transdermal drug delivery. • Raw material in the formulation is non toxic in nature. • More stable • The transethosomal drug is administrated in a semisolid form. • Avoidance of first pass metabolism • Biocompatible and Biodegradable	• Product loss during transfer from alcoholic and water media. • Skin irritation or allergic reaction on contact dermatitis. • Unsuccessful vesicle formation can Coalesce transethosomes.

Table 2. Comparison with other vesicular systems with their advantages and disadvantages.

4.3. Challenges of vesicular carriers

Though vesicular carriers are becoming popular day by day but due to chemical reactions like oxidation and hydrolysis of the phospholipid component of vesicular carrier, its stability is a matter of concern. The physical and chemical instability can be seen by events like leakage of encapsulated drug and change in vesicle size which takes place due to fusion and aggregation.

4.4. Comparison with different vesicular carriers

The comparison of nanoethosomes and transethosome with other vesicular carriers are described in **Table 2**.

5. Penetration mechanisms for ethanol-based vesicular carriers

5.1. Ethanol effect on skin

Nanoethosomes and transethosomes contains around 20–50% of ethanol [26]. The action of ethanol on the lipid layer is shown in **Figure 2** with comparison to the lipid layer where there is no ethanol present. **Figure 2B** is showing void space is created and filled with ethanol that in turn increased area per lipid molecule [27]. X-ray diffraction shows that the lipid bilayer has interdigitated Membrane leaflet which eventually leads to thinner membrane when ethanol comes in contact with the lipid bilayer. As the surface density of lipid decreases the bilayer gets thinner which leads to membrane distention. Due to presence of alcohol at the surface the change in membrane shape get accelerated. Chanturiya et al. experimentally proved that alcohol promote fusion of discontinuous membrane by breaking the single layer continuity. This study do not confirm about alcohol accelerating post fusion membrane distention [28]. The result that comes up from this demonstration is that presence of ethanol can bring about

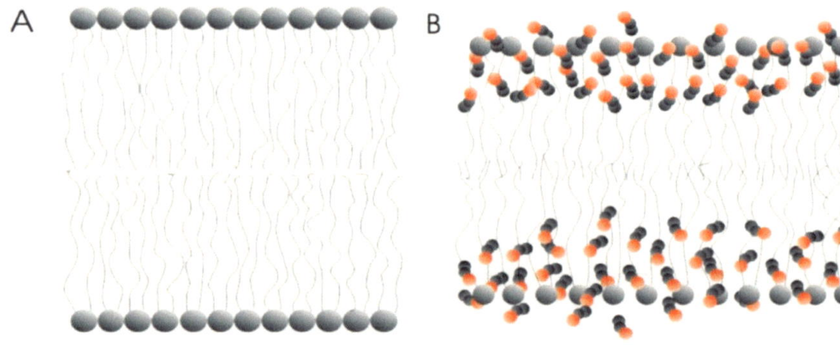

Figure 2. Schematic representation of ethanol's presence and absence on the bilayer lipid membrane: (A) representation of bilayer lipid membrane structure in the absence of ethanol; (B) presence of ethanol molecule is being represented as gray and red dots in the lipid bilayer membrane which partition into glycerol backbone and a hydrophilic head resulting in an increase in area per lipid molecule. (B) Also shows small leaflet interdigitation by representing the membrane relatively thinner as compared to (A) that shows the effect of presence of ethanol in (B).

alteration in rate of change in shape by membrane in an exocytosis manner. In this demonstration the concentration of alcohol is quite higher as compared to that which is found in the blood in case of intoxication. Ethanol does accumulate in some region of body such as striatum, brain to an extent of three times of the level that is found in blood. Clearance from alcohol from striatum is relatively slower s compared to other region of body. This characteristic may affect chronic alcoholics during an event of binge drinking as the kinetics of neurotransmission may have an implication of the said characteristics [29].

5.2. Mechanism of skin penetration through vesicular carrier

Vesicular system assists in transdermal drug delivery of molecule either by enhancing penetration of free drug component or permeation is enhanced by the component of vesicles. In some cases the transdermal drug delivery takes place by intact vesicle penetration into the skin and then through it. Vesicle get adsorb and fused with the stratum and assist the transdermal drug delivery. Ethanol a component in ethosomes and nanoethosomes act as a great permeation enhancer as it fluidizes membranous lipid bilayer along with the lipid present in stratum corneum. Liposomes contain phosphatidyl choline which is tightly packed as compared to ethosomes or nano-ethosomes where phosphatidyl choline is loosely packed. Nano ethosomal vesicles have more flexibility as compared to liposomes. Stratum corneum composed of compactly packed phospholipid, when ethanol comes in contact with it disrupts the compact packing of phospholipid and fluidizes the lipid layer. This fluidization of lipid layer is the mechanism through which drug delivery by nano-ethosomes occurs. E. Touitou et al. has carried out DSC studies for ethosomal formulation which contains 30% ethanol, 5% phospholipid and liposomes were prepared without ethanol. An investigation is carried out by M.M.A Elsayed et al. to prove that the basic mechanism of skin delivery of drug is enhancement of permeation by ethanol and flexible nature of vesicles. The investigation focused on the in-vitro profile of drug outside the vesicles, drug inside the vesicle and drug on both side of vesicle. Out of the four the formulations the drug which was present inside the vesicular carrier displayed enhanced permeation then the remaining two formulations. From this it can be concluded that presence of ethanol is not major factor of permeation, if it would have been the case then drug outside the vesicle would have shown better permeation. This also suggests that the deformable nature of vesicle assist in enhanced penetration and drug delivery of drug. Godin and Touitou [30] proved vesicle adsorption to the skin and fusion of vesicular layer with stratum corneum of skin. It is observed that the drug present in liposomal preparation is unable to penetrate into skin although the preparation gets adsorbed to the membrane. In case of ethosomal preparation the ethanol present in it gets intercalated on lipid present in stratum corneum which results in increase in membrane permeability. Ethosomes are flexible and after fusion with the membrane they successfully deliver the drug inside the cells [31]. The main parameter that defines the movement of transfersomes across the cutaneous is extent of flexibility and partition coefficient. The passage of transferosomes through the stratum corneum layer is governed by hydration force. The fluid content of stratum corneum is lower than other layer of skin due to which fluid gradient created. Cevc et al. explained the passage through skin by osmotic strength theory [14]. The active ingredient can easily release in stratum corneum and diffuse through different layer of skin and reaches blood circulation. Transferosomes pass through the intercellular space of stratum corneum by

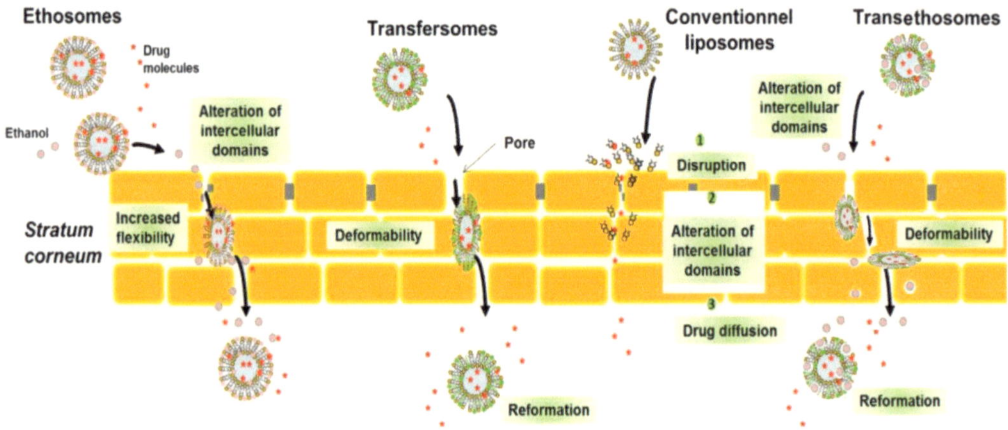

Figure 3. Schematic representation of the main permeation mechanisms of lipid-based vesicles.

deforming itself. No studies reported that transferosomes can permeate through the skin without altering its shape. The vesicular carrier transethosome makes its pathway through the stratum corneum into the deep skin layer by adhering to lipid lamella after interacting with the disturbed layer of stratum corneum. The presence of ethanol and edge activator in vesicles enhances its flexibility and fluidity and due this kind of elastic nature, vesicles can easily pass through narrow intercellular pathway. The permeation mechanism of different type of vesicular carriers is explained in **Figure 3**.

6. Method of preparation

There are four methods of preparation for nanoethosomes and transethosomes which are explain in here.

6.1. Preparation by cold method

In this method, ethanol is taken and to it phospholipid is added then by constant stirring it is dissolved at room temperature. Then to this solution propylene glycol is added and stirred vigorously. Then the solution mixture is heated up to a temperature of 30°C. Simultaneously on other hand water is being heated with up to a temperature of 30°C. Water and ethanol both solvents are used so that drug according to its affinity can dissolve in either of them. Stirring is continued to next 5 minutes. Then the suspension obtained is cooled down at maintained at room temperature. In the final step, by employing methods like extrusion or sonication, the vesicle size can be adjusted. Then the prepared ethosomal vesicles are kept in refrigerator for storage [32, 33].

6.2. Preparation by hot method

In hot method, a dispersion of phospholipid and water is subjected to heating at a temperature of 40°C. The step of heating at the same temperature is continued till colloidal solution is formed. Simultaneously in another vessel two more solvent namely glycol and ethanol is added and heated at a 40°C. When both mixtures steadily attain a temperature of 40°C then to the aqueous phase the organic phase is added. Then stirring is done up to next 5 minutes and the obtained vesicle suspension is cooled down to room temperature. Depending on the ability and affinity of drug to bind with hydrophilic and hydrophobic solvent, it either gets dissolved in water or in ethanol. The required size of ethosome vesicles can be easily prepared by using methods like extrusion or sonication [6].

6.3. Preparation by classical method

Here in this method, a mixture of ethanol, active medicaments and phospholipid is taken in such way that the active medicament and phospholipid get dissolved in ethanol. Then the solution mixture is heated by using a water bath at a temperature of about 30 ± 1°C. In the next step to solution mixture double distilled water is added with continuous stirring at a speed of 700 rpm. Then with the help of hand extruder, the obtained vesicles are homogenized for three cycles using polycarbonate membrane [34].

6.4. Preparation by mechanical dispersion method

In this method a mixture of chloroform and ethanol is taken in a round bottom flask (RBF). To the round bottom flask soya phosphatidylcholine is added and made to dissolve in the chloroform and ethanol mixture. By using rotary vacuum evaporator organic solvent is removed. This step is carried out at a temperature that is above the lipid transition temperature. The main purpose of maintaining that temperature is that at the said temperature a thin lipid film gets deposited on the surface of a round bottom flask. Then the round bottom flask is kept overnight so that trace of solvent can be obtained from the lipid film that got deposited on the round bottom flask. Then hydroethanol hydration is being done by simply rotating round bottom flask at the required temperature by employing different concentration of drug mixture [35].

7. Evaluation parameters of vesicular carriers

7.1. Morphology

Morphology defined as study of shape and size of vesicular carriers. Generally vesicular carriers are regular spherical in shape and they are physically soft and flexible and core is enclosed. On the basis of formulation, vesicular carrier may be small, unilamellar or multilamellar. With the help of microscope morphology of vesicular carrier is studied. As most of the vesicles are nano-sized so to view the morphology scanning electron microscopy is used. In addition to identification study, morphology also explains the detection the pattern of packing of particles and aggregation [36].

7.2. Particle size and size distribution

As smaller size increases the efficiency of drug delivery to the desired site, vesicles in the vesicular carriers are of nanometer to micrometer range. Uniform size is major factor to consider and it can be achieved depending on instrumentation and formulation procedures. Nanosizers are employed to measure the size and size distribution of vesicular carriers. Photon correlation spectroscopy is also used for determination of particle size [18].

7.3. Zeta potential

Distribution of charge on the surface of vesicular carrier is expressed by zeta potential. The presence of charge on the surface of nanoparticle is a major determinant of stability of the product. The presence of negative and positive charge on vesicular carrier depends upon the excipient used in the formulation. Zeta potential can be defined as the degree of electrostatic repulsion and attraction in colloidal dispersion. Zeta potential provides information regarding every components of formulation and interaction among them. It also gives information regarding surface chemistry. Zeta potential is determining factor for stability of colloidal dispersion system. It also determines the interaction between vesicles and membrane [37, 38].

7.4. Drug content

To ascertain whether the preparation content the required active ingredient in required amount in the vesicles, the vesicles are lyses so that the content is released. The released content is put into the solution then the solution is subjected to spectrophotometric analysis or chromatographic assay. Lysis of vesicles is done by solvents like isopropylalcohol, methanol, etc. [39].

7.5. Loading capacity, encapsulation efficiency, and vesicle yield

To have proper information about the drug that is actually trapped in the vesicles, entrapment is determined. For determination of entrapment, from the formed vesicles unentrapped drug is separated. Separation is done either by elution method using elution technique by the help of suitable column or by simply by the method of ultracentrifugation. Centrifugation is supposed to be done in such a controlled speed and temperature so that the vesicles do not get ruptured during the process. At end of centrifugation the supernatant produced is separated from the vesicles. Then the vesicles are treated with solvent likes triton-X. 2-propanol so that it get lysed then drug content is subjected to UV vis spectroscopy, the amount of drug entrapped is calculated [40]. The encapsulation efficiency (EE), Loading capacity (LC) and Vesicle Yield are calculated by the following formula's.

$$\mathrm{EE}\,(\%) = \frac{\mathrm{Ao} - \mathrm{Au}}{\mathrm{Ao}} \times 100 \qquad \mathrm{LC}\,(\%) = \frac{\mathrm{Ao} - \mathrm{Au}}{W} \times 100$$

$$\mathrm{Yield}\,(\%) = \frac{\mathrm{Av}}{\mathrm{Ao} + W} \times 100$$

Where Ao is the initial amount of the drug used, Au is the nonencapsulated drug, W is the amount of lipid material used in the vesicular formulation and Av is the amount of vesicular carrier produced [41].

7.6. Drug release and biophysical interactions

Drug release is dependent on many factors such as the additives used in formulation and also the physiological condition at the site of administration. As we can consider when the particle size is relatively larger and the vesicular carriers the non-flexible then their permeation across the biological membrane is hampered. Every single body part possess its particular pH, if the formulation that has to be administered in that area is in that pH range then physiological functioning is not affected but in case the formulation has pH different from the physiological pH of concerned area then physiological condition would get affected. pH can cause ionization of drugs that can result in inability of the drug to pass through the biological barrier [42, 43].

7.7. Stability

The stability of the preparation can estimate by ensuring whether there is any change in vesicle size. When stability is concerned, it is believed that homogeneous preparation is more stable as compared to heterogeneous ones. Another way of determining the stability of preparation is to study its membrane stability and molecular arrangement by X-ray scattering or differential scanning method. Study of particle size is just considered as a quality control test not a test to ascertain the internal stability of preparation. This conclusion is made as it is seen in properly lyophilized liposome, where particle size is stable but additive like cryoprotectant interfere with lipid layer molecular arrangement in bilayer membrane [44].

8. Application of nanoethosomes and transethosomes

Ethosomes and nanoethosomes have enhanced efficiency as compared to liposomes. They give 65% better results in drug delivery as compared to liposomes as they easily crosses the human skin layers. Few bioactive agents are considered to investigate the efficacy of these vesicular systems which are described in **Tables 3** and **4** [45].

8.1. Transdermal delivery of anti-fungal bioactives

To ascertain the drug delivery efficiency of vesicular carrier system for anti-fugal drugs, Bhalaria et al. conducted an experiment where they took fluconazole and prepared nano-ethosomes from them [46]. Then they took that nanoethosomal preparation and checked their efficacy in cutaneous candidiasis patients. This experiment showed positive results as the nanoethosomal preparations displayed a better clinical efficiency as compared to liposomal preparation, hydroethanolic solution and the marketed preparations of same drug. Girhepunje et al. conducted similar experiments taking ciclopiroxolamine ethosomes. Here he considered entrapment and optimized size and result of the experiment showed that due to presence of

Drug	Excipients	Sophisticated techniques used	EE (%)	Size/PDI	Animal model	Key findings
(1) Anti-fungal drugs						
Amphotericin B	Soya phosphatidylcholine, propylene glycol, ethanol	Transmission electron microscopy (TEM), confocal laser scanning microscopy (CLSM)	71.56	218.4 ± 2.9 nm/ 0.451 ± 0.03	—	Drug loaded nanoethosomes showed high drug entrapment, greater penetration power, and high stability compared to liposomes
Clotrimazole	Soya phosphatidyl choline (Phospholipon 90 H), ethanol	TEM, atomic force microscopy (AFM), FT-IR spectroscopy	68.73 ± 1.4	%/132 ± 9.5 nm/ 0.027 ± 0.011	Sprague Dawley rats	Nanoethosomes showed high drug entrapment, enhanced transdermal permeation flux, and *in-vitro* anti-fungal activity compared to ultradeformable liposomes; along with high zone of inhibition compared to marketed formulation
Clotrimazole	Cavamax (W6, W7, and W8), propylene glycol, ethanol, triethanolamine, iso-propylmyristate	TEM, CLSM	98.42 ± 0.15	202.8 ± 4.8 nm/ 0.113 ± 0.024	Wistar albino rats	Cavamax W7 composite ethosomal gel showed high drug permeation flux, deeper penetration in epidermis and high anti-fungal activity against *Candida albicans* and *Aspergillus niger* compared to normal ethosomal gel
Griseofulvin	Phospholipon 90G, Carbopol 980 NF, ethanol	TEM, fluorescence microscopy, reverse phase HPLC	72.94 ± 0.80	148.5 ± 0.48 nm/ 0.203	Laca mice	Griseofulvin-loaded Ethosomes completely cured fungal infection in guinea pigs in 8 days upon twice daily topical applications
(2) Cardiovascular drugs						
Minoxidil	Phospholipon 90, ethanol, phosphotungstic	TEM, CLSM, HPLC, 31P-NMR	83 ± 6	153 ± 15 nm/–	Male albino mice	Prepared nanoethosomal formulation at 2% phosphatidylcholine and 30% ethanol showed rapid enhancement in transdermal permeability of compared hydroethanolic or phospholipid ethanolic solution of minoxidil
Valsartan	Phospholipon 90G, ethanol, cholesterol	TEM, CLSM, HPLC	89.34 ± 2.54	209 ± 15 nm/–	Wistar albino rats	Results of study showed penetration of nanoethosomes in deeper skin layers compared to conventional liposomes and 3.03 times increase in bioavailability compared to oral suspension of valsartan

http://dx.doi.org/10.5772/intechopen.81152

Drug	Excipients	Sophisticated techniques used	EE (%)	Size/PDI	Animal model	Key findings
(3) Antiviral drugs						
Lopinavir	Phospholipon 90 H, cholesterol, ethanol	TEM, fluorescence microscopy, HPLC	79.6 ± 4.1	112.8 ± 12.4 nm/ 0.131 ± 0.008	Wistar rats	Fluorescence study revealed better disposition of ethosomal carrier in rat skin compared to niosomes; but, *in-vivo* extent of absorption was high in case of niosomal carrier system
Hepatitis B surface antigen-	Soya phosphatidylcholine, Span 80, ethanol	Flow-cytometric analysis, spectral bioimaging	—	—	—	Nanoethosomes showed high internalizing capacity and immunogenicity compared to elastic liposomes following transcutaneous route
Indinavir	Soya phosphatidylcholine, ethanol	TEM, SEM, HPLC	96.71 ± 1.4	147 ± 4.5 nm/ 0.12 ± 0.03	Human cadaver skin	Nanoethosomes showed greater permeation of drug through human cadaver skin along with shortest lag time compared to conventional liposomes
(4) Anti-inflammatory drugs						
Triptolide	Dipalmitoylphosphatidyl choline, cholesterol, ethanol	HPLC	98.8 ± 4.7	123.1 ± 8.6 nm/ 0.335	Sprague Dawley rats	Nanoethosomal formulation showed highest *in-vitro* accumulation of Triptolide in skin and significant reduction in erythema *in-vivo* in rat model
Aceclofenac	Soybean phosphatidylcholine, isopropyl alcohol	Scanning electron microscopy (SEM)	95.7	0.696 μm/–	—	Nanoethosomal formulation showed very high transdermal flux and high stability for 45 days compared to an ethanolic drug solution
Diclofenac sodium	Soya lecithin, cholesterol, ethanol	Photon correlation spectroscopy	51.72 ± 4.36	202 ± 20.6 nm/ 0.34	Sprague Dawley rats	Nanoethosomal formulation showed high permeation through rat skin and permeability coefficient of nanoethosomes was 15-folds higher than conventional liposomes
Ketoprofen	Soya phosphatidyl choline, cholesterol, ethanol	TEM, CLSM, HPLC	78.7 ± 4.9	120.3 ± 6.1 nm/–	Adult Chinese	Nanoethosomal formulation showed high transdermal flux and high *in-vitro*

Drug	Excipients	Sophisticated techniques used	EE (%)	Size/PDI	Animal model	Key findings
					female skin	penetration compared to hydroethanolic solution of drug through human skin
(5) Miscellaneous bioactive materials						
Glimepiride	Phospholipon 90 G, propylene glycol, cholesterol, ethanol	SEM, TEM, HPLC, CLSM	99.89%	93 nm/–	Male Wistar rats	*In-vivo* study of ethosomes in human volunteers showed extended drug release behavior and lower maximum drug plasma level when used in the form of transdermal films
Apigenin	Lipoid S 75, propylene glycol, ethanol	TEM, HPLC	85.21 ± 3.97	36.61 ± 1.78 nm/–	Sprague Dawley rats	Apigenin loaded nanoethosomes showed effective reduction of cyclooxygenase-2 levels in mouse skin inflammation induced by ultraviolet B (UVB) light compared to liposomes/deformable liposomes
Tacrolimus	Lipoid S 100, absolute ethanol	TEM, HPLC	79.8 ± 1.6	76.3 ± 0.5 nm/ 0.26 ± 0.01	BALB/c mice	Tacrolimus loaded nanoethosomes showed higher encapsulation efficiency, lower vesicle size, and skin penetration compared to conventional liposomes with cholesterol
Paclitaxel	Phospholipon 90G, absolute	HPLC, TEM, cell cycle analysis and apoptotic determination	82.00 ± 1.78	240.0 ± 61.48 nm/ 0.145 ± 0.047	Adult human skin	Paclitaxel loaded nanoethosomes showed improved penetration capacity through stratum corneum epidermal membrane model and increased antiproliferative activity in squamous cell carcinoma model as compared to the free drug solution
5–Aminolevulinic acid (ALA)	Phosphatidyl ethanolamine, ethanol	Colorimetry, CLSM, HPLC	—	—	—	CLSM study showed depth of penetration of nanoethosomes up to 80 μm in murine skin and penetration studies showed 26-folds increase in transdermal flux of nanoethosomes compared to plain ALA solution

Table 3. Applications of nanoethosomes for transdermal delivery of various classes of drugs.

Drug	Excipients	Sophisticated Techniques used	EE (%)	Size/PDI	Animal model	Key findings
Voriconazole	Lipoid S100, cholesterol, Tween80, taurocholic acid sodium, ethanol	TEM, HPLC	96.6 ± 2.7	191.9 ± 41.5 nm/–	Male albino mice	Prepared transethosomes showed high elasticity, high *in-vitro* skin permeation, and high *in-vivo* skin deposition of voriconazole compared to nanoethosomes and conventional liposomes
Ketorolac tromethamine	Phospholipon 90G, sodium deoxycholate, propylene glycol, ethanol	TEM, FT-IR	82.08 ± 4.5%/	180 ± 70 nm/–	Male albino rats	Transethosomes showed 3-fold more elasticity compared to ethosomes and transethosomal gel 3-fold increase in transdermal flux compared to conventional ethosomes
Vitamin E	Soybean phosphatidyl choline, sodium cholate, ethanol	TEM, HPLC	76.689 ± 2.942	154.73 ± 1.89 nm/ 0.428 ± 0.020	Pig ear skin	For transdermal flux and stability, order obtained was: transethosomes (TE) > ethosomes (E) ≥ transferosomes (T) for vitamin E
Caffeine	Soybean phosphatidyl choline, Sodium cholate, ethanol	TEM, HPLC	3.376 ± 0.812	116.60 ± 2.25 nm/ 0.133 ± 0.015	Pig ear skin	For transdermal flux and stability, order obtained was: transethosomes (TE) > ethosomes (E) ≥ transferosomes (T) for caffeine
Griseofulvin	Phospholipon 90G, Carbopol 980 NF,	TEM, HPLC fluorescence microscopy, reverse phase	72.94 ± 0.80	148.5 ± 0.48 nm/ 0.203	Laca mice	Griseofulvin-loaded ethosomes completely cured fungal infection in guinea pigs in 8 days upon twice daily topical applications

Table 4. Applications of transethosomes for transdermal delivery of some miscellaneous drugs.

45% ethanol there is higher level of entrapment and vesicles formed are of optimized size [47]. **Table 3** provides information regarding few of the researches that has been conducted on nanoethosomal drug delivery of anti-fungal class of drug.

8.2. Transdermal delivery of anti-inflammatory bioactives

To have an idea about the efficacy of ethosomal preparation in delivering anti-inflammatory drug Paolino et al. conducted an investigative experiment on few human volunteers taking ethosomes entrapped with ammonium glycyrrhizinate. The ethosomal preparation which was having an ethanol content about 45% and having a lesser lecithin content gave better results both in *in-vitro* and *in-vivo* consideration. In case of in vitro it showed enhanced percutaneous permeation, better tolerability of skin, and in vivo consideration showed enhanced anti-inflammatory activity in human volunteers. Nanoethosomes being smaller in size and having higher content of ethanol displayed better entrapment efficiency. Brief information has been given in **Table 3** regarding transdermal delivery of anti-inflammatory drug [48].

8.3. Transport of drug with action on cardiovascular system

To ascertain the extent of delivery of cardiovascular drug from transdermal system of drug delivery Touitou et al. investigated the efficiency of nanoethosomes filled with minoxidil. The nanoethosomes that were prepared with 2% of phosphatidylcholine and 30% of ethanol displayed a relatively increased permeability when compared with the formulation of hydroethanolic and phospholipid minoxidil. In another experiment Ahad et al. took valsartan and investigated the penetration capability of the nanoethosomes containing valsartan in the skin of Wistar albino rats. The results were amazing as there was increased penetration into deeper layers of skin when compared with liposomal preparation of same drug and it also shows increased bioavailability when compared with oral route of administration. In addition to this Bhosale and Avachat documented an increased antihypertensive action in Wistar albino rats when given transdermally as compared with oral administration of same [49]. **Table 3** shows role of nanoethosomes in antihypertensive drug delivery.

8.4. Transport of bioactive agent with antiviral activity

Nanoethosomes of lamivudine is been prepared by Jain et al. to evaluate the efficacy of transdermal delivery of antiviral drugs. The nanoethosomal preparation showed 25 times better penetration of drug through as compared to a simple solution. T-lymphocytes showed increased uptake ability for nanoethosomes compared to free drug solution [33]. Few more examples regarding transdermal drug delivery of antiviral drug is given in **Table 3**.

8.5. Delivery of miscellaneous bioactives

Nanoethosomes were compared with hydroethanolic and liposomal preparation, for that Dayan & Touitou prepared a nanoethosomes that was loaded with trihexyphenidyl HCl and result that came were really great as nanoethosomes showed better transdermal permeation than both the above mentioned preparation [50]. The penetration of nanoethosomes was deeper as compared to conventional liposomes. Dubey et al. studied melatonin loaded nanoethosomes in cadaver skin of human and are compared with liposomes. Result showed high mobility of drug through skin in case of nanoethosomes. **Table 3** provides brief information about nanoethosomes for delivery of various types of drugs [35].

9. Patent related to nanoethosomes

First patent related to nanoethosomes granted in 1986 by Prof. Elka Touitou of Hebrew University School of Pharmacy, Jerusalem. Descriptions of few patents regarding transdermal drug delivery of nanoethosomes are given in **Table 5.**

Title of patent	Brief description	Inventors	Patent number
Ethosome preparation of male hormone medicaments and its preparation method	This invention describes the preparation technique of ethosomes loaded with male hormone used to treat various male diseases like male sterility, endocrine erectile dysfunction, and male climacteric syndrome	Guan Yan Min, MengShu, Li Jianxin, Dan	CN102406605 A
Progesterone ethosome, and preparation method and application there of	This invention describes a method of encapsulation of progesterone (0.1–1%) in ethosomes for treatment of secondary amenorrhea, dysfunctional bleeding, and premenstrual syndrome	Zhang Shu, Deng Hong, Lin Huaqing, Zhang Xiaoling	CN102397255 B
Transdermal composition for treating pain	This invention describes ethosomal composition for transdermal delivery for treatment of pain; the present invention can be used to treat different type of pain like muscular, nociceptive and neuropathic in origin	Moheb Maalawy	WO2015123750 A1
Preparation method of lidocaine ethosome	This invention discloses a method of preparation of lidocaine ethosomes using lecithin and ethanol as major constituent; prepared ethosomes showed entrapment up to 80.93% and good skin compatibility	Liang Ju, Wu Wenlan, Li, Miao Juan, Wei Xuefeng, Chen Shan, Wang Xiaotaro	CN102688194 B
Daptomycin ethosome preparation	This invention describes preparation method of daptomycin ethosomes using 1 mg daptomycin, 10–20 mg lecithin, 0.6–0.8 ml ethanol, and balance of water; the ethosomes show low preparation cost and high stability	Lee Chong, Liu Ha, YanqiKun, Wang Xiaoying, Chen Po	CN103006562 B
Phenasteride gel preparation	This invention discloses preparation method of phenasteroid using 0.5–4% phospholipid and their dispersion in carbomer (0.25–1.5%) gel for topical application	Liang Wen- right, RaoYuefeng	CN1555804 A
Bullatacin ethosome gel and preparation method thereof	This invention describes method of preparation of ethosomal gel using Brad he octyl, phospholipid, low molecular weight alcohol, cholesterol, stabilizer, and antioxidant; size of ethosome is 30–400 nm	Tan Jianping, Jiang Lixin, often calm, Zhou Zhiwen	CN102552147 B
Acyclovir ethosome and preparation method thereof	This invention discloses acyclovir loaded ethosomes with improved stability by addition of polyethylene glycol or chitosan for percutaneous administration	Wuxue Wen, Xiong Yan	CN102133183 B
Ethosomes preparation of antimycotics pharmaceutical and method for preparing the same	This invention discloses an ethosomal preparation loaded with anti-fungal drug containing 1–8% phospholipid, 20–45% ethanol, and 40.9–78.9% of water	Liu Liping, Li Yimin, ShenMing- high, six Jiang Hu, Yang Jin	CN101273971 A

Title of patent	Brief description	Inventors	Patent number
Clotrimazole ethosomes for preventing and curing weaning rabbit dermatomycosis and preparation method thereof	This invention describes the composition and method of preparation of ethosomes loaded with clotrimazole having 3% of lecithin and 1% of clotrimazole by weight	Liu Man, Mou special, Liming Yong	CN104873465 A

Table 5. Description of patents related to nanoethosomes for transdermal drug delivery.

10. Conclusion

The work presented here is an overview on one of the current novel drug delivery device named as vesicular carrier. For researchers in the field of novel drug delivery vesicular carrier has become an area of interest which makes the future of vesicular carrier application bright in field of therapeutics and drug delivery. As vesicular carrier has an inert ability to better factors like solubility, penetration, uptake as well as it provides a better carrier facility to ensure the stability of various types of drugs and proteins, this makes it bankable delivery system of bioactive agents. In addition to this vesicular system is compatible with both hydrophilic as well as hydrophobic drug and easy encapsulate them. It also encapsulate herbal bio agent and ensure their stability. These said characteristics makes vesicular carrier system a promising option in the field pharmaceutical nanotechnology and herbal medicines. Vesicular carrier system has few thing as drawbacks like instability, relatively smaller short shelf life or difficulty to reach the target. All the drawbacks can be overcome by few techniques like providing appropriate storage condition to maintain stability, giving a polymeric coating to the preparation or conjugating the preparation with suitable ligands. To ascertain or assess the vesicular carrier stability and acceptability said parameters can be employed.

Author details

Koushlesh Kumar Mishra[1]*, Chanchal Deep Kaur[2], Shekhar Verma[3], Anil Kumar Sahu[1], Deepak Kumar Dash[1], Pankaj Kashyap[1] and Saraswati Prasad Mishra[1]

*Address all correspondence to: koushleshmishra@gmail.com

1 Royal College of Pharmacy, Raipur, Chhattisgarh, India

2 Shri Rawatpura Sarkar Institute of Pharmacy, Kumhari, Chhattisgarh, India

3 Pt. Deendayal Upadhyay Memorial Health Sciences and Ayush University, Raipur, Chhattisgarh, India

References

[1] Almandil NB. Healthcare professionals' awareness and knowledge of adverse drug reactions and pharmacovigilance. Saudi Medical Journal. 2016;**37**:1359-1364. DOI: org/10.15537/smj.2016.12.17059

[2] Robert A, Freitas L Jr. Bioscience. In: Nanomedicine, Basic Capabilities. Vol. I. USA: Landes Bioscience; 1999

[3] Godin B, Touitou E. Mechanism of bacitracin permeation enhancement through the skin and cellular membranes from an ethosomal carrier. Journal of Controlled Release. 2004;**94**(2–3):365-379

[4] Barry B. Breaching the skin's barrier to drugs. Nature Biotechnology. 2004;**22**(2):165-167

[5] Honeywell NPL, Bouwstra JA. Vesicles as a tool for transdermal and dermal delivery. Drug Discovery Today: Technologies. 2005;**2**(1):67-74

[6] Pandey V, Golhani D, Shukla R. Ethosomes: Versatile vesicular carriers for efficient transdermal delivery of therapeutic agents. Drug Delivery. 2015;**22**(8):988-1002. DOI: 10.3109/10717544.2014.889777

[7] Pirvu DC, Hlevca C, Ortan A, Prisada R. Elastic vesicles as drugs carriers through the skin. Farmácia. 2010;**58**(2):128-136

[8] Gregoriadis G, Florence AT. Liposomes in drug delivery. Clinical, diagnostic and ophthalmic potential. Drugs. 1993;**45**(1):15-28

[9] Sharma A, Sharma SU. Liposomes in drug delivery: Progress and limitations. International Journal of Pharmaceutics. 1997;**154**(2):123-140

[10] Schreier H, Bouwstra JA. Liposomes and niosomes as topical drug carriers: Dermal and transdermal drug delivery. Journal of Controlled Release. 1994;**30**(1):1-15

[11] Rai K, Gupta Y, Jain A, Jain SK. Transfersomes: Self-optimizing carriers for bioactives. PDA Journal of Pharmaceutical Science and Technology. 2008;**62**:362-379

[12] Regnier V, De Morre N, Jadoul A, Préat V. Mechanisms of a phosphorothioate oligonucleotide delivery by skin electroporation. International Journal of Pharmaceutics. 1999;**184**:147-156

[13] Fahy E, Subramaniam S, Murphy R, Nishijima M, Raetz C, Shimizu T, et al. Update of the LIPID MAPS comprehensive classification system for lipid. Journal of Lipid Research. 2009;**50**(Supplement):S9-S14

[14] Cevc G. Transfersomes, liposomes and other lipid suspensions on the skin: Permeation enhancement, vesicle penetration, and transdermal drug delivery. Critical Reviews in Therapeutic Drug Carrier Systems. 1996;**13**(3–4):257-388. DOI: 10.4103/2231-4040.85524

[15] Honeywell-Nguyen PL, Bouwstra JA. The *in vitro* transport of pergolide from surfactant based elastic vesicles through human skin: A suggested mechanism of action. Journal of Controlled Release. 2003;**86**(1):145-156. DOI: 10.1016/S0168-3659(02)00415-7

[16] Trotta M, Peira E, Carlotti ME, Gallarate M. Deformable liposomes for dermal administration of methotrexate. International Journal of Pharmaceutics. 2004;**270**(1–2):119-125. DOI: 10.1016/j.ijpharm.2003.10.006

[17] Song CK, Balakrishnan P, Shim CK, Chung SJ, Chong S. A novel vesicular carrier, transethosome, for enhanced skin delivery of voriconazole: Characterization and *in vitro/in vivo* evaluation. Colloids and Surfaces. B, Biointerfaces. 2012;**92**:299-304. DOI: 10.1016/j.colsurfb.2011.12.004

[18] Mbah CC, Builders PF, Attama AA. Nanovesicular carriers as alternative drug delivery systems: Ethosomes in focus. Expert Opinion on Drug Delivery. 2014;**11**(1):45-59. DOI: 10.1517/17425247.2013.860130

[19] Touitou E. Composition of applying active substances to or through the skin. International Patent: International Publication Number US 5716638. 1996

[20] Lopez-Pinto JM, Gonzalez-Rodriguez ML, Rabasco AM. Effect of cholesterol and ethanol on dermal delivery from DPPC liposomes. International Journal of Pharmaceutics. 2005;**298**(1):1-12. DOI: 10.1016/j.ijpharm.2005.02.021

[21] Zhou Y, Wei Y, Liu H, Zhang G, Wu X. Preparation and in vitro evaluation of ethosomal total alkaloids of Sophora alopecuroides loaded by a transmembrane pH-gradient method. AAPS PharmSciTech. 2010;**11**:1350-1358

[22] Verma P, Pathak K. Therapeutic and cosmeceutical potential of ethosomes: An overview. Journal of Advanced Pharmaceutical Technology & Research. 2010;**1**(3):274-282

[23] Vijay Kumar SK, Parthiban S, Kumarsenthil PG, Mani Tamiz T. ETHOSOME-A new trends In vesicular approaches for topical drug delivery. Asian Journal of Research in Pharmaceutical Sciences and Biotechnology. 2014;**2**(1):23-30

[24] Shahwal V, Samnani A, Dubey B, Bhowmick M. Ethosomes:An overview. International Journal of Biomedical and Advance Research. 2011;**2**:161-168

[25] Patel S. Ethosomes: A promising tool for transdermal delivery of drug. Pharmalnfo.Net. 2007;**5**(3):38-43

[26] Touitou E, Dayan N, Bergelson L, Godin B, Eliaz M. Ethosomes—Novel vesicular carriers for enhanced delivery: Characterization and skin penetration properties. Journal of Controlled Release. 2005;**65**:403-418

[27] Lauer AC, Ramachandran C, Leib LM, Niemiec S, Simon ND. Effect of ethanol on membrane order: Fluorescence Weiner, targeted delivery to the pilosebaceous units via studies. Annals of the New York Academy of Sciences. 1987;**492**:125-133

[28] Bergelson LD, Molotkovsky JM, Manevich YM, Touitou L. A clinical evaluation of a novel liposomal carrier specific fluorescent probes in studies of biological mem-for acyclovir in the topical treatment of recurrent herpesbranes. Chemistry and Physics of Lipids. 1985;**37**: 165-161

[29] Gillet A, Compère P, Lecomte F, Hubert P, Ducat E, Evrard B, et al. Liposome surface charge influence on skin penetration behaviour. International Journal of Pharmaceutics. 2011;**411**:223-231. DOI: 10.1016/j.ijpharm.2011.03.049

[30] Godin B, Touitou E. Critical Reviews in Therapeutic Drug Carrier Systems. 2003;**20**(1): 63-102

[31] Mezei M, Gulusekharam V. Liposomes—A selective drug delivery system for the topical route of administration. Life Sciences. 1980;**26**:1473-1477

[32] Touitou E. Composition for applying active substances to or through the skin. International Patent: International Publication Number US 5716638 1998

[33] Jain S, Tiwary AK, Sapra B, Jain NK. Formulation and evaluation of ethosomes for transdermal delivery of lamivudine. AAPS PharmSciTech. 2007;**8**(4):E111. DOI: 10.1208/pt0804111

[34] Manosroi A, Jantrawut P, Khositsuntiwong N, Manosroi W, Manosroi J. Novel elastic nano-vesicles for cosmeceutical and pharmaceutical applications. Journal of the Science Faculty of Chiang Mai University. 2009;**36**(2):168-178

[35] Dubey V, Mishra D, Jain NK. Melatonin loaded ethanolic liposomes: Physicochemical characterization and enhanced transdermal delivery. European Journal of Pharmaceutics and Biopharmaceutics. 2007;**67**(2):398-405. DOI: 10.1016/j.ejpb.2007.03.007

[36] Maestrelli F, Capasso G, Gonzalez-Rodriguez ML, Rabasco AM, Ghelardini C, Mura P. Effect of preparation technique on the properties and in vivo efficacy of benzocaine-loaded ethosomes. Journal of Liposome Research. 2009;**19**(4):253-260

[37] Radomska-Soukharev A. Stability of lipid excipients in solid lipid nanoparticles. Advanced Drug Delivery Reviews. 2007;**59**:411-418

[38] Severino P, Szymanski M, Favaro M, Azzoni AR, Chaud MV, Santana MHA. Development and characterization of a cationic lipid nanocarrier as nonviral vector for gene therapy. European Journal of Pharmaceutical Sciences. 2015;**66**:78-82

[39] Mbah C, Builders P, Nzekwe I, Kunle O, Adikwu M, Attama A. Formulation and in vitro evaluation of pH-responsive ethosomes for vaginal delivery of metronidazole. Journal of Drug Delivery Science and Technology. 2014;**24**(6):565-571

[40] Jain S, Sapre R, Tiwary AK, Jain NK. Proultraflexible lipid vesicles for effective transdermal delivery of levonorgestrel: Development, characterization, and performance evaluation. AAPS PharmSciTech. 2005;**6**(3):E513-E522

[41] Nikpoor AR, Tavakkol-Afshari J, Gholizadeh Z, Sadri K, Babaei MH, Chamani J. Nanoliposome-mediated targeting of antibodies to tumors: IVIG antibodies as a model. International Journal of Pharmaceutics. 2015;**495**:162-170

[42] Almeida AJ, Florindo HF. Nanostructures overcoming the nasal barrier: Physiological considerations and mechanistic issues. In: Alonso MJ, Csaba NS, editors. Nanostructured Biomaterials for Overcoming Biological Barriers. Cambridge, MA: RSC Publishing; 2012. pp. 117-132

[43] Salama AH, Aburahma MH. Ufasomes nano-vesicles-based lyophilized platforms for intranasal delivery of cinnarizine: Preparation, optimization, ex-vivo histopathological safety assessment and mucosal confocal imaging. Pharmaceutical Development and Technology. 2014;**21**(6):706-715. DOI: 10837450.2015.1048553

[44] Stark B, Pabst G, Prassl R. Long-term stability of sterically stabilized liposomesby freezing and freeze-drying: Effects of cryoprotectants on structure. European Journal of Pharmaceutical Sciences. 2010;**4**:546-555

[45] Touitou E, Dayan N, Bergelson L, Godin B, Eliaz M. Ethosomesnovel vesicular carriers for enhanced delivery: Characterization and skin penetration properties. Journal of Controlled Release. 2010;**65**(3):403-418. DOI: 10.1016/S0168-3659(99)00222-9

[46] Bhalaria MK, Naik S, Misra AN. Ethosomes: A novel delivery system for antifungal drugs in treatment of topical fungal disease. Indian Journal of Experimental Biology. 2009;**47**(5): 368-375

[47] Girhepunje K, Pal R, Gevariya H, Behera A, Thirumoorthy N. Ethosomes: A novel vesicular carrier for enhanced dermal delivery of Ciclopirox Olamine. Der Pharmacia Lettre. 2010;**2**(1):360-367

[48] Paolino D, Lucania G, Mardente D, Alhaique F, Fresta M. Ethosomes for skin delivery of ammonium glycyrrhizinate: *In vitro* percutaneous permeation through human skin and *in vivo* skin anti-inflammatory activity on human volunteers. Journal of Controlled Release. 2005;**106**(1–2):99-110

[49] Ahad A, Aqil M, Kohli K, et al. Enhanced transdermal delivery of an anti-hypertensive agent via nanoethosomes: Statistical optimization, characterization and pharmacokinetic assessment. International Journal of Pharmaceutics. 2013;**443**(1–2):26-38. DOI: 10.1016/j.ijpharm.2013.01.011

[50] Dayan N, Touitou E. Carriers for skin delivery of trihexyphenidyl HCl ethosomes vs. liposomes. Biomaterials. 2001;**21**(18):1879-1885. DOI: 10.1016/S0142-9612(00)00063-6

Chapter 3

Nano-Antimicrobial Solutions Using Synthetic-Natural Hybrid Designs

Teodora Mocan, Ofelia Mosteanu, Cristian T. Matea,
Teodora Pop, Nadim Al-Hajjar, Cosmin Puia,
Luminita Furcea, Cristina Bura and Lucian Mocan

Additional information is available at the end of the chapter

http://dx.doi.org/10.5772/intechopen.81156

Abstract

Nanotechnology potential in antimicrobial therapy is increasingly demonstrated by various data. Results reveal antibacterial properties, comparable to that of conventional antibiotics. Working on parallel experiments, researchers continue to bring evidence demonstrating age-old-recognized antibacterial properties of various natural components of plant and animal origin. Later years brought an increasing trend for combining synthetic and natural composition in new constructs. The tendency aims to bring more on different essential aspects, such as active substance release, improvement of antibacterial effect, and up-regulation of the mechanisms at the structure-cell interface. Present chapter structures the up-to-date achievements in the field, including the concept of design, biological effects, benefits, mechanisms, and limitations of the field. Also, expected future research directions are to be discussed.

Keywords: antimicrobial, synthetic, natural, nanotechnology, antibacterial

1. Introduction

Microbial infections represent a major health problem, being responsible for more than 16 million cases of pathology-related death cases per year [1]. The impact is increased by the appearance of multidrug-resistant bacteria, a mounting tendency, responsible for both acute and chronic forms of clinical presentations of such infections. The need for urgent generation of new, valid therapy solutions, capable of eluding the resistance mechanisms, has been increasingly high during late years. Nanotechnology potential in antimicrobial therapy is increasingly demonstrated by various data. Nanoparticles such as zinc oxide, silver, aluminum oxide, iron oxide, copper, titanium dioxide, and silicon dioxide have been successfully tested by various research groups [1]. Results reveal antibacterial properties, as demonstrated by testing strains of *Escherichia coli* [2], *Staphylococcus aureus* [3], *Staphylococcus epidermidis* [4], or *Pseudomonas aeruginosa* [5]. Working on parallel experiments, researchers continue to bring evidence demonstrating age-old recognized antibacterial properties of various natural components of plant and animal origin. The presence of phenols and phenolic acids [6], quinones [7], flavonoids [8], tannins [9], terpenoids [10], alkaloids [11], lectins, and other polypeptides [12, 13] in the composition provides bactericidal or bacteriostatic effect by activating various biological mechanisms. Present chapter summarizes the most recent achievements in new designs of therapeutic solutions involving both natural components as well as laboratory processing and/or synthetic components. Also, some of the most common antimicrobial mechanisms of those structures are to be analyzed.

2. Green synthesis of nanoparticles exhibiting antimicrobial role

The idea of nanoparticle synthesis using green technology represents one of the first, beginning trends in joining the two different domains: nanotechnology and natural extract chemistry. Although the final composition of the nanoparticles designed this way does not necessarily include high concentrations of natural extracts, the concept of green design aims to diminish the risk of possible chemical traces resulting from nanoparticle synthesis in the final product. Reducing or stabilizing agents could be good examples of such traces. In the new green synthesis concept, any traces, if present, would be a part of a natural compound with rather beneficial than dangerous effects. One such report is the synthesis of silver nanoparticles using *Acorous calamus* rhizome extract. The extract was prepared starting from *Acorous calamus* rhizome powder, using a mixing (100 mL soluble distilled water) technique, associated with heating (60°C, 10 min) and filtering procedures. Manufacturing of nanoparticles was further performed using a 5:1 ratio mixing of aqueous $AgNO_3$ solution and natural extract, respectively, followed by room temperature, 24 h of incubation. Centrifugation (18,000 rpm), repetitive washing followed by room temperature, and drying were used by researchers to collect the nanoparticles. Complete characterization including spectral (UV-Vis, SEM/EDX, FTIR) techniques, hydrodynamic measurements (DLS) as well as simultaneous application of thermogravimetric and differential scanning calorimetric techniques (TGA-DSC analysis) certified the synthesis of nanoparticles. The manufactured nanostructures have revealed strong antibacterial effect against *Bacillus subtilis*, *Staphylococcus aureus* as well as *Bacillus cereus*. Disk diffusion technique revealed 1.5, 1.7, and 1.6 cm if inhibition zone, compared to the streptomycin standard responsible for 3.4, 3.1, and 2.6 cm of inhibition performed against streptomycin control. Similarly, growth kinetic studies analyzing the effect of a 40 μg/mL concentration of synthetized nanoparticles on *Escherichia coli* showed significant inhibition within the log phase (active phase) of bacterial growth, a demonstration of antibacterial activity [14]. Similar results were reported by other groups. One such research team used *Boerhavia diffusa* plant extract as a reducing agent and tested the newly synthetized silver nanoparticles for their antibacterial role. The whole-plant extract of *Boerhavia diffusa* involved collection, washing of plant, drying, followed by Soxhlet apparatus-based extraction and power formulation by reducing under pressure. Dilution of the extract (500 mg in 100 mL distilled water) and mixing with $AgNO_3$ solution (10 mL prepared extract solution: 90 mL 0.1 M $AgNO_3$) followed by heating, (100°C, continuous stirring, 15 min), discarding of supernatant, collecting, and drying of sediment were used for the synthesis of the nanoparticles. SDR, SEM, TEM, as well as UV-VIS analyzes demonstrated the formation of silver nanoparticles. Three selected fish pathogen strains were used, namely *Aeromonas hydrophila, Flavobacterium branchiophilum,* and *Pseudomonas fluorescens* and the determination of minimum inhibitory concentration was performed. The MIC values for *Flavobacterium branchiophilum, Aeromonas hydrophila,* and *Pseudomonas fluorescens* were 3.12, 25, and 50 μg/mL, respectively. Although values differed from one bacterial strain to another, the designed silver nanoparticles revealed similar diameter of inhibition zone with that of Rifampicin for concentration values of 50 μg/mL (15, 14, 12 mm, respectively, for *Flavobacterium branchiophilum, Aeromonas hydrophila, Pseudomonas fluorescens*). [15]. Similarly, callus extracts of *Sesuvium portulacastrum* L. from tissue cultures were successfully used for the generation of silver nanoparticles. Preparation of callus was performed following a previously reported technique [16]. For the synthesis of silver nanoparticles, callus extraction steps (grinding of 20 g fresh callus, boiling for 5 min, centrifugation of 3000 rpm), mixing with $AgNO_3$ solution, incubation (dark), and stabilization with polyvinyl alcohol were carried out. The antibacterial activity was found to be efficient as demonstrated by clinical microbial strain testing with inhibition zones ranging from 11 to 17 mm (*Staphylococcus aureus, Pseudomonas aeruginosa, Micrococcus luteus, Listeria monocytogenes,* and *Klebsiella pneumoniae*) [17]. *E. coli*-directed antimicrobial activity was also documented by disk diffusion method in the case of a carob leaf extract-mediated synthesis of silver nanoparticles. Extract was performed using a consecutive step procedure including washing, sun-drying, cutting followed by boiling in distilled water, filter separation, and centrifugation (1200 rpm, 5 min) for heavy metal removing. Synthesis of nanoparticles was carried out by mixing 5 mL aqueous extract with 100 mL of 1×10^{-3} M $AgNO_3$ solution. Several techniques were involved in characterization of nanomaterial UV-VIS and FTIR spectral techniques, x-ray diffractometry, and SEM, all of which demonstrated a fast and efficient formation of silver nanoparticles. The effect has been reported to be superior to standard antibiotic, with a minimum inhibitory concentration for silver nanoparticles of 0.5 μg/L, while the standard antibiotic calculated value was 0.6 mg/L [18]. Moreover, unique designs based on silver nanoparticles, such as silk fibroin-silver nanoparticle composites, have also been reported. The natural polymer *Bombyx mori* was used as a scaffold for synthesis of silver nanoparticles in situ, under the effect of light. The synthesis included preparation of silk-fibroin solution involving degumming steps (0.5 wt% $NaHCO_3$, 100°C, 30 min), dissolving step (9.3 mol-L LiBr solution, 60°C), dialyze step, centrifugation (6000 rpm, 5 min), and collection of supernatant. Next, composite synthesis was carried out, including mixing of $AgNO_3$ powders (5–8 mg) and 1 wt% silk-fibroin solution (5 mL), followed by UV light exposure and incubation (room temperature, 24 h). The construct demonstrated biofilm-destructive properties as well as direct antibacterial effects against methicillin-resistant *Staphylococcus aureus*. The minimal inhibitory concentration was reported to be 19.2 mg/L for silver nanoparticles within the composite material [19].

However, not only silver nanoparticles have been reported to be successfully synthetized using green technologies. One report provided evidence of triangular gold nanoparticles synthesis by using extract of *Aloe vera* plant. 6 mL of 0–3 M aqueous $HAuCl_4$ solution were mixed with distinct volumes (0.5–4 mL) of *Aloe vera* extract (obtained by butting and boiling procedures), and volume of each sample was completed up to 10 mL. The authors provide evidence of possible modulatory effect of the *Aloe vera* concentration on optical and morphological properties of gold nanoparticles. Addition of *Aloe vera* (in different amounts) can vary the size of gold nanoparticles from 50 to 350 nm. Also, possible shapes of nanoparticles include spherical, triangular, and hexagonal or rod-like patterns. The team demonstrates strong near-infrared absorbance, suggesting a good potential for hyperthermia-modulated applications, such as anticancer or antimicrobial effects [20]. Similarly, gold nanoparticles were published to have been synthetized using *Memecylon edule* leaf extract. The experiment passed through a first step of *Memecylon edule* extract, using washing, drying under dark, cutting into smaller parts, powdering (mixer), boiling (20 g powder, 100 mL water, 5 min), incubation (dark, 30°C), and filtering. In a consecutive step, a bioreduction process was carried out involving aqueous leaf extract in different concentrations (15, 10, and 5 mL, respectively) and $HAuCl_4$ solutions (1 mM, 10 mL). The gold nanoparticles presented a plate-like morphology and various shapes: triangular, spherical, tetraedrical. The dimension ranges between 20 and 35 mm. Each shape was demonstrated to induce distinct optical properties, with decisive importance on the future antimicrobial plasmonic resonance-based applications [21]. Recently, the diversity of structures and concepts of materials have been increasing. Nanosize crystals of ZnO have been manufactured using *Nephelium lappaceum* L. peel extracts. Procedures of natural extract preparation involved washing and cutting of peels, followed by oven-drying, (50°C), boiling (3 g dried rambutan, 1:2 ratio of ethanol:water for 10 min), and filtering. The technology, involving zinc-ellagate complex formation resulted in coating of cotton fabric with ZnO nanocrystals. Synthesis of ZnO nanocrystals was carried out by slow addition of 10 mL of rambutan peel extract in 50 mL of 0.1 M of $Zn(NO_3)_2.6H_2O$ sol (stirring, 80°C, 2 h), followed by several centrifugation steps, oven-drying (40°C, 8 h), and calculation (muffle furnace, 450°C). Material has been added with ZnO nanocrystals (12 × 12 cm dimension, 2% ZnO, 1% citric acid solution, 5 min,) further processed using the padding mangle run (15 m/min, 15 kgf/cm^2), and was subject to thermal drying (3 min, 140°C). Removal of unbound crystals, and soap traces and final drying ended the experimental protocol. Such material demonstrated both Gram-negative (*E. coli*) as well as Gram-positive (*S. aureus*) bacteria. According to disk diffusion results, the largest inhibition area corresponded to *S. aureus* (23 mm in diameter), while *E. coli* revealed 18.5 mm diameter inhibition [22]. Similar cotton fibers loaded with silver nanoparticles were designed by using natural tree leaves *Ficus benghalensis* and *Eucalyptus citriodora*. The extract preparation protocol included intense washing (15 min, 15°C), drying, preparation of leaf broth solution (100 mL water with 2, 4, or 6 g of leaves), heating of solution (100°C), extraction (30 min), and filtering. Synthesis of nanoparticles was performed by mixing of natural extract (2, 4, or 6 g in 5 mL) with 1 mM aqueous $AgNO_3$ solution (1:1 volume ratio). Immersion of cotton fibers in the Mixt solution (shaker, 1000 rpm, room temperature, 24 h) and drying ended the protocol. The authors have demonstrated efficient antimicrobial effect against *E. coli* in case of 2% leaf extract, even after repetitive water washing of treated fabric at different time intervals (5, 10, 15, 30 min, 1, 3, 5, 10, 15, and 24 h) [23]. Also, recently, a new waterborne paint additive with antimicrobial properties has been reported. The authors reported the generation of zinc oxide nanoparticles (partially covered with silver) by means of flame spray pyrolysis, followed by powder dispersion through stirring and sonication. Characterization of obtained product included specific surface area assessment, transmission electron microscopy analyzes, x-ray fluorescence testing, and dynamic light scattering measurements, demonstrating the structure, conformation, and dimensions of nanoparticles included in the product. Testing of antimicrobial effect was performed using a standardized method (ISO 22196:2011, modeled by Japanese standard JIS Z 2801:2000). In brief, survival counts were estimated after spreading of different concentrations of ZnO-Ag nanopowder (0.1, 0.2, 0.3, and 0.4%) and ZnO nanopowder on solidified plates containing 10^9 colony forming units of each of the microorganism (tryptone soy agar, 0.6% (W/v) yeast extract, nutrient agar). Results showed significant antimicrobial effect against *Staphylococcus aureus, Salmonella* spp., *Listeria monocytogenes, Bacillus subtilis,* and *Pseudomonas* spp. with an inhibition zone of >5 mm [24].

A special class of green synthesis designs involves the use of alternative sources for reduction and stabilizing agents, apart from plant or animal origin. Using bacterial, actinomycete, yeast, or fungal strains for providing the necessary material for green synthesis is more recently an interesting technological solution. The use of *Candida guilliermondii* was reported recently for silver as well as for gold nanoparticle production. The nanoparticles demonstrated efficiency against *Staphylococcus aureus*, unlike the chemically synthetized silver and gold nanoparticles who demonstrated no antimicrobial effect. The results demonstrate the enhancing of antimicrobial properties due to green synthesis protocol [25]. Intracellular synthesis of gold nanoparticles by using a special strain of *Rhodococcus* species was reported. Experimental protocol included isolation of *Rhodococcus* sp., maintenance (potato-dextrose agar slants), monthly subculturing, and preservation. Mycelia were produced by growing of actinomycete in MGYP medium, separation (centrifugation 200 rpm, 27°C, 96 h), and washing. Gold nanoparticles were isolated by resuspension of mycelia in aqueous $HAuCl_4$ solution (10^{-3} M). Successful biotransformation was certified by UV-VIS spectra, TEM, and XRD analyzes [26]. Also, *Bacillus licheniformis* has been successfully used for synthesis of silver nanocrystals. Isolation of bacteria (collection, incubation 37°C, 48 h) and characterization of isolates were followed by addition of $AgNO_3$ (1 mM) solution to 2 g wet biomass previously inoculated with bacterial isolate [27]. For another report, the synthesis was carried out by using fungal strains, such as *Fusarium acuminatum*. After isolation from infected ginger and characterization of extract, fabrication of biomass was carried out (incubation of fungal culture at 28°C in potato sucrose broth, inoculation onto flasks, agitation, and filtration). Synthesis was carried out by mixing $AgNO_3$ solution with the filtrate for a final concentration of 1 mM, followed by 2 h incubation. Such nanoconstructs, resulted from mycosynthesis and validated by UV-VIS and TEM analysis, demonstrated efficiency against *S. aureus* (17 mm inhibition), *S. epidermidis, S. typhi*, or *E. coli* (10 mm) in the exact mentioned order (from highest to lowest efficiency) [28].

3. Nanoencapsulation and microencapsulation of natural compounds designed for antibacterial applications

3.1. Cyclodextrin encapsulation

Increasing the efficiency of natural compounds as well as diminishing their drawbacks, such as limited bioavailability or excessive rate of release, has been one major and constant research topics during late years. Several practical approaches have been designed. Polymer-based nanoparticles as well as naturally derived nanocarriers were the most common experimental trends [29]. Phenolic compounds as well as the specific component piperine are known to be present in black pepper oleoresin. Researchers have started to improve their biological interaction properties by approaching the encapsulation in cyclodextrins. Although the capsules are relying on a natural-based material, their laboratory processing and characterizing the newly designed construct represented an important research step. Testing data also revealed not only higher antioxidant activity for the encapsulated extract, but also more efficient antibacterial effect as compared to nonencapsulated compound. Data revealed that lower concentrations are needed for inhibiting the growth of the Salmonella strain used for evaluation and demonstrated that designed formulation is able to improve the antimicrobial effect of the natural extract [30]. β-Cyclodextrin encapsulation has also been selected by Mourtzinos et al. for optimization of olive leaf natural extract properties. The active component, oleuropein has been already demonstrated to exert anticancer [31] effects, inhibitory efficiency against certain human pathogens such as Mycoplasma [32], as well as to provide antioxidant protection [33], and the obtained formulation offered protection for the natural extract toward better biological effect. Similarly, Dima et al. used an extract coming from *Coriandrum sativum* L. seeds and structured a formulation by β-cyclodextrin encapsulation. Testing revealed an intense inhibition of 2,2-diphenyl-1-picrylhydrazyl radicals for 30 μg/mL. The newly designed capsular formulation has proven to have important stronger antioxidant activity as compared to widely accepted standards (ascorbic acid, butylated hydroxytoluene). Also, antimicrobial and antifungal activities have been reported [34].

3.2. Complex coacervation

A distinct attempt of providing improved properties for natural extracts by hybrid processing was involving complex coacervation. The extract used was that of propolis, already known as a natural-source food additive. Isolated pectin and soy protein were used as encapsulation material. Although the compounds used in encapsulation were of natural origin, isolation of compounds and the complex coacervation protocol represented a step forward in improving the properties of nanomaterials by encapsulation. The authors have demonstrated the technology to generate a stable, alcohol-free agent in a powder formulation that elicits controlled release properties, but also demonstrated antimicrobial activity against *Staphylococcus aureus* [35].

3.3. Polymer-based encapsulation and liposomes

However, most researchers have focused toward synthetic, polymer-based systems as well as liposomes.

The need for packaging food using materials with antibacterial properties motivated the work of a research team who designed nanocapsules with cinnamaldehyde. The capsules were designed as lipid bilayers of polydiacetylene-N-hydroxysuccinimide (PDA-NHS) nanoliposomes. Immobilization on glass slide was further performed and this type of product demonstrated significant antibacterial activity against *E. coli* as well as *Bacillus cereus* in (2.56 log10 and 1.59 log10 CFU/mL, respectively; reduction in 48 h) [36]. The efficacy of liposomes containing cinnamon natural extracts against methicillin-resistant *Staphylococcus aureus* (MRSA) was also demonstrated in a recent article and was appreciated as satisfactory by the team. As colony forming unit determination reveals, such formulation could offer high efficiency against MRSA biofilms on various classes of substrates, from steel, nonwoven fabrics, gauze, and up to nylon membranes. The formulation was demonstrated to augment stability of antibacterial effect and to prolong the period of action [37]. Similarly, Fennel extract was encapsulated by another center, in the attempt to create food additives able to exert antimicrobial role on the fish meat (carp species). The extract demonstrated antioxidant effects, as well an antibacterial effect as revealed by the microbial count. The efficacy of the liposome-encapsulated form proved superior in terms of oxidative deterioration to tissues and reducing of microbial colonization. The formulation also provided extended shelf life following treatment of carp fillet [38]. Another recent report also demonstrated superior antioxidant and antimicrobial properties of Thymus species extracts. The team obtained an enriched antioxidant activity and antimicrobial effect of the liposomes containing extracts coming from the four selected species of Thymus as compared to the extract alone [39]. Similar thyme extract was encapsulated into liposomes by researchers and the effect on microbial colonization and oxidative injury on silver carp was analyzed compared to controls using a 15 day monitorization period. The growth inhibition of *E. coli* O_{15}:H_7 was demonstrated, and the total bacterial estimation in the food had proved superior in the encapsulated formulation as compared to natural extract, therefore presenting the designed liposomes suitable for carp meat food additives [40]. Driven conclusions were equally sustained by a distinct research group, who finds the phytosomes as suitable for drug and food applications, their stability, physicochemical properties, and antibacterial efficiency being dependent of specific method of synthesis. The liposomal encapsulation is considered as preserving the activity of bioactive components as compared to water solution, this particularity being caused by the elevated water solubility and reduced lipid solubility [41].

A more extensive study tested various encapsulation designs for active components such as lysozyme, nisin as well as various herbs and spice extracts, including liposomal, chitosan as well as polysaccharide encapsulation. The advantage of liposomal formulation could come from their higher stability compared to chitosan encapsulation. Antimicrobial activity against both positive and negative of Gram bacteria was efficient and stable for a minimum of 1 month. Due to the controlled release possibility derived from the formulation concept, the authors indicate a large potential for applications under hydrogel form with embedded capsules containing natural extracts [42].

Recently, the synthesis protocols became more oriented toward complex structures, such as polymer-lipid nanoparticles. One of the most robust designs is represented by a core-shell concept, presenting a polymeric core, a lipid shell with embedded active substance, and protected by polyethylene-glycol moieties for immunoreactivity reduction [43]. The advantages of such structures come from increased stability, morphological and structural integrity, low risk of damage during storage, controlled release features, elevated biocompatibility, and bioavailability. Both the polymeric and the lipidic component can be built using not only artificial, but also using natural sources, such as chitosan or natural fatty acids and represent the next generation of materials directed toward antimicrobial applications [44].

4. Nanoparticles functionalized with natural biomolecules

Not all research groups have followed the encapsulation trend. A part of the research teams have focused on direct attachment of biologically active, natural origin molecules onto the surface of metal nanoparticles. One such design was the synthesis of catechin-Cu nanoparticles. By joining two elements with already known antibacterial effect, the newly formed compound was reported to induce a 3 h-death rate of up to 90 and 85% of *S. aureus* and *E. coli*, respectively, as assessed by means of the live/dead bacterial viability kit by the authors [45]. Similarly, iron oxide nanoparticles were functionalized with natural source gallic acid. The resulting construct was demonstrating significant antibacterial effect against *E. coli*, *S. aureus*, and *B. subtilis*, comparable with that exerted by ampicillin or streptomycin [46]. Also, chitosan, a natural polysaccharide, was demonstrated as presenting improved efficiency when binded to copper or zinc nanoparticles, and the effect has been published to be proportional to the level of zeta potential [47].

Silver nanoparticles were also reported to have been successfully functionalized with glucosamine, a natural sugar. The newly constructed compound presented high antimicrobial efficiency. Both *Klebsiella pneumoniae* and *Bacillus cereus* were more sensitive to the functionalized as compared to pristine AgNps, as demonstrated by minimum inhibitory concentration determination [48]. Research has been advancing toward ore and more complex designs. In another publication, a crosslinked chitosan-coated Ag-loaded nano-SiO_2 composite was reported to exert a good antimicrobial activity against *S. aureus* as well as *E. coli*, and the authors demonstrate the synergic action of all included components in the structure as being responsible for improved effect [49]. Another biofilm-destructive solution was that of polysaccharide-bound silver nanoparticles. Green synthesis of caboxy-methyl-tamarind, polysaccharide-capped silver nanoparticles was performed, and the newly designed construct has demonstrated inhibitory effects against *E. coli* and *B. subtilis* growth. The obtained effect could be efficient against bacterial biofilm formation and consolidation [50].

5. Mechanisms underlying the antimicrobial effect of natural-synthetic hybrid materials

Although consistent efforts have been made for development of hybrid, natural-synthetic designs, as well as testing their antimicrobial effects, there is still limited data regarding the exact mechanisms involved in the obtained antimicrobial effects. However, the natural compound in the construct can be considered as an important contributor in the final bacterial inhibition mechanism. The most important antimicrobial mechanisms involved in natural extract action, along with studies detailing the effect, are summarized below.

5.1. Membrane permeabilization, membrane potential alterations, and cellular component leakage

One of the most incriminated antimicrobial mechanisms used by natural extracts involves the functional and structural integrity of the membrane. Alteration of bacterial membrane potential demonstrated by Saritha et al. is a study focused on different extracts. *Leucas aspera, Hemidesmus indicus, and Plumbago zeylanica* ethanolic extracts revealed different mechanisms of membrane functional attack. While data on the ethanolic extracts of *Hemidesmus indicus* and *Plumbago zeylanica* revealed disruption of membrane continuity with leakage of cellular content and consecutive alteration of membrane potential, extract of *Leucas aspera* demonstrated functional alteration properties, with limited anatomical destruction consecutive to exposure. The latter was found to generate inner membrane alterations with preservation of outer membrane continuity, therefore lacking complete permeabilization. The effects were studied on *E. coli*. Authors provided evidence on green emission fluorochrome leakage as well as electron microscopy evidences of membrane blebbing with release of cellular contents. Such events could be possibly explained by the presence of flavonoid and phenol antioxidant molecules in the extracts, known to exert a detergent-like effect. Moreover, the antimicrobial effects were proven to be dependent on concentration and time [51]. Similarly, morphological changes such as cell membrane tearing with interference with the cell's survival were found by researchers as a mechanism used by *Polygonum cuspidatum*, a Chinese age-old therapeutic plant. The extract induced significant morphological changes such as: membrane rupturing, and content release into the exterior all followed by cell death, as images provided by scanning electron microscope have revealed [52].

Detailed evidences of protein leakage were brought by a distinct research group, while testing the effects of *Cocos nucifera* extract. The effects after bacterial exposure were analyzed from the minimal inhibitory concentration, protein potassium ions leakage from cells as well as nucleotide release following membrane permeabilization. Results demonstrate significant antimicrobial effects. Calculated MIC was ranging between 0.39 and 12.5 mg/mL. The time-kill analyze identifies 15 min as the minimal time interval for bacterial death following exposure, with 27.8% rate of death. For a concentration of 1 × MIC, protein leakage at the identified time point was ranging between 3.56 and 19.08 μg/mL, potassium ions leaked between 0.182 and 0.379 mg/mL while the nucleotides ranged between 0.609 and 2.446 μg/mL [53]. In a similar manner, the assessment of the effects exerted by *Veronica montana* L. extract was performed by researchers. Various bacterial strains, including Gram-positives and Gram-negatives were tested, by monitoring their sensitivity to exposure to extract. The most sensitive strain has been *L. monocytogenes,* and the mechanism suggested by testing data was direct lysis of pathogenic cytoplasmic membrane [54]. Also, another research group has studied the effects of monocaprylate, as a naturally generated molecule. The team focused on the mechanisms underlying the death induced by monocaprylate on different strains, such as *E. coli*, *Staphylococcus xylosus*, and *Zygosaccharomyces bailii*. Cell morphology and content, as well as continuity of membrane were examined. Different methods, such as atomic force microscopy and propidium iodide staining, were used to depict the mechanisms. Also, by means of quartz crystal microbalance measurements, the authors have measured the concentration of monocaprylate in the samples. Based on obtained data and theoretical considerations, the authors have reasoned that the sensitivity of the membrane itself plays a role in the molecule-membrane interaction. Lipidic componence, fluidity of membrane as well as the sphericity of the membrane may play an important role. It has been demonstrated that the destructuring of membrane by the chosen testing molecule is done by increasing the amount of membrane and the fluidity level [55]. Moreover, in a recent study, intensive oxygen reactive species generation, with consecutive membrane destabling and protein leakage, was found following exposure of *Salmonella typhimurium* (as well as other strains) to the methanolic extract of *Scutellaria barbata* (*S. barbata*). The mechanisms resulted in a 24.7% death rate in the exposed bacteria following 40 min of treatment The results add a new physiopathological element to the mechanistic chain responsible for antimicrobial effects, by demonstrating the involvement of oxidative stress in the early onset of membrane alterations and content release responsible for bacterial death [56].

5.2. Alterations in regulation of gene expression

The release of bacterial cell content as a result to treatment-induced permeabilization is preceded by enhanced expression of different proteins. Yong et al. have identified several distinct proteins with up-regulated expression following medicinal plant exposure, namely chaperonin (60 kDa), flagellin, triacylglycerol lipase, outer membrane protein A, N-acetylmuramoyl-L-alanine amidase, 30S ribosomal protein s1, and stringent starvation protein A. The paper suggests common antibacterial routes for different natural antimicrobial treatments [57].

Similarly, evidences provided by El-Hamid et al. support the conclusion of inducing down-regulation of quorum-sensing system. Altering bacterial communication, exerted by plant natural therapies was demonstrated by qRT-PCR and was reported to be induced by down-regulation of quorum-sensing already established genes [58]. Also, transcription processes as well as replication of nucleic acids (DNA/RNA) were reported [59].

5.3. Metabolic alterations

Besides the already discussed mechanisms, a recent paper has discussed the addition of metabolic-induced alterations by exposure to natural extracts. The mechanisms identified by the authors were respiratory enzymatic inhibition, inducement of oxidative stress, heat-shock state, and forcement of bacterial acute stringent response. The ATP level tends to decrease in the cell, as demonstrated by the *E. coli* strain O_{157}:H_7 used by the authors, following exposure to different natural-source extracts such as: thymol, carvacrol, (þ)-carvone, or trans-cinnamaldehyde [59].

5.4. Effects induced by nanoparticles

The antimicrobial effect of particular nanomaterials represents a complex interaction of distinct effects. Modulation of effects could theoretically come from the cell internalization of free ions resulting from the nanomaterials, cell-nanostructure interaction, and physical properties of the nanostructures such as dimension, morphology, or surface charge. Due to the large area provided by the surface of nanoparticle, the different chemical nature of nanostructures and the final effects are hard to predict and therefore represent a serious research aim for each individual type of nanomaterial [60]. Among antibacterial applications, silver nanoparticles represent a major fraction of tested materials due to widely accepted and traditionally known effects of silver. For this nanomaterial, in particular, effects are mainly due to silver ion uptake, resulting in DNA toxicity and membrane damage [60].

6. Drawbacks, limitations, and future research trends

The mounting of medicinal resistance in bacteria and the constant changes in bacterial mechanisms against antibiotics trigger the need for different solutions, which would include a natural-based antimicrobial component. Present limitations, however, come from the little interest of pharmaceutical companies in integrating nature-provided elements into their fabrication process. Extraction and testing by specialized companies could provide an additional solution for antibacterial treatment, and should be focused on age-old validated plants used in traditional medicine [61].

The future of research within the discussed topic is dependent on improved mechanistic understanding at the interface between material and bacterial cell, as well as more in depth knowledge on nanomaterials and their specific behavior in different conditions. The more knowledge acquired, the more complex and tailored the structure of the future constructs will be. Concepts of future structures are becoming themselves a research topic necessary for generation of better nano-antimicrobial constructs [62].

7. Conclusions

The advances in nano-antimicrobials based on synthetic-natural (hybrid) designs join the achievements of two domains already demonstrating promising data for future biocide agents. Up-to-date literature suggests acceleration along the path of generating new antibacterial agents, capable to respond to the problem of severe resistance to conventional antibiotics and holding good promises for the future of the domain. Most concepts of synthesis protocols demonstrate practical efficiency, comparable with the standard recommended antibiotic treatment. However, while most polymer-based and liposomal designs were meant for textile and packaging treatment, functionalization of nanoparticles with naturally active compounds seems to suit direct antimicrobial treatment better, including the possibility for adding topics in human-intend applications. Distinctly, capsular products benefit from digestive transit protection of active components, thus making them perfect for oral administration. Concept design results in specific tailoring of final product; therefore, the choice of technology and prototype remains to be made based on the final desired application.

Acknowledgements

This work was supported by the Romanian National Authority for Scientific Research and Innovation, CNCS-UEFISCDI, project numbers PN-III-P2-2.1-BG-2016-0446, PN-III-P1-1.1-PD-2016-1831, and PN-III-P1-1.1-TE-2016-2161.

Author details

Teodora Mocan[1,2*], Ofelia Mosteanu[1,2], Cristian T. Matea[1,2], Teodora Pop[1,2], Nadim Al-Hajjar[1,2], Cosmin Puia[1,2], Luminita Furcea[1,2], Cristina Bura[1,3] and Lucian Mocan[1,2]

*Address all correspondence to: teodora_mocan@yahoo.com

1 "Iuliu Hatieganu" University of Medicine and Pharmacy, Cluj-Napoca, Romania

2 "Prof. Dr. Octavian Fodor" Regional Institute of Gastroenterology and Hepatology, Cluj-Napoca, Romania

3 "Dr. Constantin Opris" Emergency County Hospital, Baia Mare, Romania

References

[1] Seil JT, Webster TJ. Antimicrobial applications of nanotechnology: Methods and literature. International Journal of Nanomedicine. 2012;**7**:2767-2781

[2] Pal S, Tak YK, Song JM. Does the antibacterial activity of silver nanoparticles depend on the shape of the nanoparticle? A study of the Gram-negative bacterium *Escherichia coli*. Applied and Environmental Microbiology. 2007;**73**(6):1712-1720

[3] Tran N, Mir A, Mallik D, Sinha A, Nayar S, Webster TJ. Bactericidal effect of iron oxide nanoparticles on *Staphylococcus aureus*. International Journal of Nanomedicine. 2010;**5**:277-283

[4] Taylor EN, Webster TJ. The use of superparamagnetic nanoparticles for prosthetic biofilm prevention. International Journal of Nanomedicine. 2009;**4**:145-152

[5] Morones JR, Elechiguerra JL, Camacho A, Holt K, Kouri JB, Ramírez JT, et al. The bactericidal effect of silver nanoparticles. Nanotechnology. 2005;**16**(10):2346

[6] Brantner A, Maleš Ž, Pepeljnjak S, Antolić A. Antimicrobial activity of *Paliurus spina*-christi Mill.(Christs Thorn). Journal of Ethnopharmacology. 2002;**52**(1):119-122

[7] Kazmi MH, Malik A, Hameed S, Akhtar N, Ali SN. An anthraquinone derivative from *Cassia italica*. Phytochemistry. 1994;**36**(3):761-763

[8] Tsuchiya H, Sato M, Miyazaki T, Fujiwara S, Tanigaki S, Ohyama M, et al. Comparative study on the antibacterial activity of phytochemical flavanones against methicillin-resistant *Staphylococcus aureus*. Journal of Ethnopharmacology. 1996;**50**(1):27-34

[9] Haslam E. Natural polyphenols (vegetable tannins) as drugs: Possible modes of action. Journal of Natural Products. 1996;**59**(2):205-215

[10] Tassou C, Drosinos F, Nychas G. Effects of essential oil from mint (*Mentha piperita*) on *Salmonella enteritidis* and *Listeria monocytogenes* in model food systems at 4 and 10°C. The Journal of Applied Bacteriology. 1995;**78**(6):593-600

[11] Omulokoli E, Khan B, Chhabra S. Antiplasmodial activity of four Kenyan medicinal plants. Journal of Ethnopharmacology. 1997;**56**(2):133-137

[12] Zhang Y, Lewis K. Fabatins: New antimicrobial plant peptides. FEMS Microbiology Letters. 1997;**149**(1):59-64

[13] Gupta A, Landis RF, Rotello VM. Nanoparticle-based antimicrobials: Surface functionality is critical. F1000Res. 2016;**5**:364-374

[14] Nakkala JR, Mata R, Gupta AK, Sadras SR. Biological activities of green silver nanoparticles synthesized with *Acorous calamus* rhizome extract. European Journal of Medicinal Chemistry. 2014;**85**:784-794

[15] Kumar PV, Pammi S, Kollu P, Satyanarayana K, Shameem U. Green synthesis and characterization of silver nanoparticles using *Boerhaavia diffusa* plant extract and their anti bacterial activity. Industrial Crops and Products. 2014;**52**:562-566

[16] Murashige T, Skoog F. A revised medium for rapid growth and bio assays with tobacco tissue cultures. Physiologia Plantarum. 1962;**15**(3):473-497

[17] Nabikhan A, Kandasamy K, Raj A, Alikunhi NM. Synthesis of antimicrobial silver nanoparticles by callus and leaf extracts from saltmarsh plant, *Sesuvium portulacastrum* L. Colloids and Surfaces B: Biointerfaces. 2010;**79**(2):488-493

[18] Awwad AM, Salem NM, Abdeen AO. Green synthesis of silver nanoparticles using carob leaf extract and its antibacterial activity. International Journal of Industrial Chemistry. 2013;**4**(1):29

[19] Fei X, Jia M, Du X, Yang Y, Zhang R, Shao Z, et al. Green synthesis of silk fibroin-silver nanoparticle composites with effective antibacterial and biofilm-disrupting properties. Biomacromolecules. 2013;**14**(12):4483-4488

[20] Chandran SP, Chaudhary M, Pasricha R, Ahmad A, Sastry M. Synthesis of gold nanotriangles and silver nanoparticles using *Aloe vera* plant extract. Biotechnology Progress. 2006;**22**(2):577-583

[21] Elavazhagan T, Arunachalam KD. Memecylon edule leaf extract mediated green synthesis of silver and gold nanoparticles. International Journal of Nanomedicine. 2011;**6**: 1265-1278

[22] Yuvakkumar R, Suresh J, Nathanael AJ, Sundrarajan M, Hong S. Novel green synthetic strategy to prepare ZnO nanocrystals using rambutan (*Nephelium lappaceum* L.) peel extract and its antibacterial applications. Materials Science and Engineering: C. 2014;**41**:17-27

[23] Ravindra S, Mohan YM, Reddy NN, Raju KM. Fabrication of antibacterial cotton fibres loaded with silver nanoparticles via "Green Approach". Colloids and Surfaces A: Physicochemical and Engineering Aspects. 2010;**367**(1-3):31-40

[24] Tornero AF, Blasco MG, Azqueta MC, Acevedo CF, Castro CS, López SR. Antimicrobial ecological waterborne paint based on novel hybrid nanoparticles of zinc oxide partially coated with silver. Progress in Organic Coatings. 2018;**121**:130-141

[25] Mishra A, Tripathy SK, Yun S. Bio-synthesis of gold and silver nanoparticles from *Candida guilliermondii* and their antimicrobial effect against pathogenic bacteria. Journal of Nanoscience and Nanotechnology. 2011;**11**(1):243-248

[26] Ahmad A, Senapati S, Khan MI, Kumar R, Ramani R, Srinivas V, et al. Intracellular synthesis of gold nanoparticles by a novel alkalotolerant actinomycete, *Rhodococcus* species. Nanotechnology. 2003;**14**(7):824

[27] Kalimuthu K, Babu RS, Venkataraman D, Bilal M, Gurunathan S. Biosynthesis of silver nanocrystals by *Bacillus licheniformis*. Colloids and Surfaces B: Biointerfaces. 2008;**65**(1): 150-153

[28] Ingle A, Gade A, Pierrat S, Sonnichsen C, Rai M. Mycosynthesis of silver nanoparticles using the fungus *Fusarium acuminatum* and its activity against some human pathogenic bacteria. Current Nanoscience. 2008;**4**(2):141-144

[29] Esfanjani AF, Jafari SM. Biopolymer nano-particles and natural nano-carriers for nano-encapsulation of phenolic compounds. Colloids and Surfaces B: Biointerfaces. 2016;**146**:532-543

[30] Teixeira BN, Ozdemir N, Hill LE, Gomes CL. Synthesis and characterization of nano-encapsulated black pepper oleoresin using hydroxypropyl beta-cyclodextrin for antioxidant and antimicrobial applications. Journal of Food Science. 2013;**78**(12):N1913-N1920

[31] Saenz M, Garcia M, Ahumada M, Ruiz V. Cytostatic activity of some compounds from the unsaponifiable fraction obtained from virgin olive oil. Il Farmaco. 1998;**53**(6):448-449

[32] Furneri PM, Marino A, Saija A, Uccella N, Bisignano G. In vitro antimycoplasmal activity of oleuropein. International Journal of Antimicrobial Agents. 2002;**20**(4):293-296

[33] Andreadou I, Iliodromitis EK, Mikros E, Constantinou M, Agalias A, Magiatis P, et al. The olive constituent oleuropein exhibits anti-ischemic, antioxidative, and hypolipidemic effects in anesthetized rabbits. The Journal of Nutrition. 2006;**136**(8):2213-2219

[34] Dima C, Cotarlet M, Tiberius B, Bahrim G, Alexe P, Dima S. Encapsulation of coriander essential oil in beta-cyclodextrin: Antioxidant and antimicrobial properties evaluation. Romanian Biotechnological Letters. 2014;**19**(2):9128-9140

[35] Nori MP, Favaro-Trindade CS, de Alencar SM, Thomazini M, de Camargo Balieiro, Julio C, et al. Microencapsulation of propolis extract by complex coacervation. LWT–Food Science and Technology. 2011;**44**(2):429-435

[36] Makwana S, Choudhary R, Dogra N, Kohli P, Haddock J. Nanoencapsulation and immobilization of cinnamaldehyde for developing antimicrobial food packaging material. LWT–Food Science and Technology. 2014;**57**(2):470-476

[37] Cui H, Li W, Li C, Vittayapadung S, Lin L. Liposome containing cinnamon oil with antibacterial activity against methicillin-resistant *Staphylococcus aureus* biofilm. Biofouling. 2016;**32**(2):215-225

[38] Mazandrani HA, Javadian S, Bahram S. The effect of encapsulated fennel extracts on the quality of silver carp fillets during refrigerated storage. Food Science & Nutrition. 2016;**4**(2):298-304

[39] Gortzi O, Lalas S, Chinou I, Tsaknis J. Reevaluation of antimicrobial and antioxidant activity of *Thymus* spp. extracts before and after encapsulation in liposomes. Journal of Food Protection. 2006;**69**(12):2998-3005

[40] Javadian SR, Shahosseini SR, Ariaii P. The effects of liposomal encapsulated thyme extract on the quality of fish mince and *Escherichia coli* O_{157}:H_7 inhibition during refrigerated storage. Journal of Aquatic Food Product Technology. 2017;**26**(1):115-123

[41] Karimi N, Ghanbarzadeh B, Hamishehkar H, Keivani F, Pezeshki A, Gholian MM. Phytosome and liposome: The beneficial encapsulation systems in drug delivery and food application. Applied Food Biotechnology. 2015;**2**(3):17-27

[42] Matouskova P, Marova I, Bokrova J, Benesova P. Effect of encapsulation on antimicrobial activity of herbal extracts with lysozyme. Food Technology and Biotechnology. 2016;**54**(3):304-316

[43] Hadinoto K, Sundaresan A, Cheow WS. Lipid–polymer hybrid nanoparticles as a new generation therapeutic delivery platform: A review. European Journal of Pharmaceutics and Biopharmaceutics. 2013;**85**(3):427-443

[44] Chan JM, Zhang L, Yuet KP, Liao G, Rhee J, Langer R, et al. PLGA–lecithin–PEG core–shell nanoparticles for controlled drug delivery. Biomaterials. 2009;**30**(8):1627-1634

[45] Li H, Chen Q, Zhao J, Urmila K. Enhancing the antimicrobial activity of natural extraction using the synthetic ultrasmall metal nanoparticles. Scientific Reports. 2015;**5**:11033

[46] Shah ST, A Yehya W, Saad O, Simarani K, Chowdhury Z, A Alhadi A, et al. Surface functionalization of iron oxide nanoparticles with gallic acid as potential antioxidant and antimicrobial agents. Nanomaterials. 2017;**7**(10):306

[47] Du W, Niu S, Xu Y, Xu Z, Fan C. Antibacterial activity of chitosan tripolyphosphate nanoparticles loaded with various metal ions. Carbohydrate Polymers. 2009;**75**(3):385-389

[48] Veerapandian M, Yun K. Synthesis of silver nanoclusters and functionalization with glucosamine for glyconanoparticles. Synthesis and Reactivity in Inorganic, Metal-Organic, and Nano-Metal Chemistry. 2010;**40**(1):56-64

[49] Mei N, Xuguang L, Jinming D, Husheng J, Liqiao W, Bingshe X. Antibacterial activity of chitosan coated Ag-loaded nano-SiO_2 composites. Carbohydrate Polymers. 2009;**78**(1):54-59

[50] Sanyasi S, Majhi RK, Kumar S, Mishra M, Ghosh A, Suar M, et al. Polysaccharide-capped silver nanoparticles inhibit biofilm formation and eliminate multi-drug-resistant bacteria by disrupting bacterial cytoskeleton with reduced cytotoxicity towards mammalian cells. Scientific Reports. 2016;**6**:24929

[51] Saritha K, Rajesh A, Manjulatha K, Setty OH, Yenugu S. Mechanism of antibacterial action of the alcoholic extracts of *Hemidesmus indicus* (L.) R. Br. ex Schult, *Leucas aspera* (Wild.), *Plumbago zeylanica* L., and *Tridax procumbens* (L.) R. Br. ex Schult. Frontiers in Microbiology. 2015;**6**:577

[52] Su P, Yang C, Yang J, Su P, Chuang L. Antibacterial activities and antibacterial mechanism of *Polygonum cuspidatum* extracts against nosocomial drug-resistant pathogens. Molecules. 2015;**20**(6):11119-11130

[53] Akinpelu DA, Alayande KA, Aiyegoro OA, Akinpelu OF, Okoh AI. Probable mechanisms of biocidal action of *Cocos nucifera* Husk extract and fractions on bacteria isolates. BMC Complementary and Alternative Medicine. 2015;**15**(1):116

[54] Stojković DS, Živković J, Soković M, Glamočlija J, Ferreira IC, Janković T, et al. Antibacterial activity of *Veronica montana* L. extract and of protocatechuic acid incorporated in a food system. Food and Chemical Toxicology. 2013;**55**:209-213

[55] Hyldgaard M, Sutherland DS, Sundh M, Mygind T, Meyer RL. Antimicrobial mechanism of monocaprylate. Applied and Environmental Microbiology. 2012;**78**(8):2957-2965

[56] Tang Q, Kang A, Lu C. Phytochemical analysis, antibacterial activity and mode of action of the methanolic extract of *Scutellaria barbata* against various clinically important bacterial pathogens. International Journal of Pharmacology. 2016;**12**(2):116-125

[57] Yong A, Ooh K, Ong H, Chai T, Wong F. Investigation of antibacterial mechanism and identification of bacterial protein targets mediated by antibacterial medicinal plant extracts. Food Chemistry. 2015;**186**:32-36

[58] El-Hamid MIA. A new promising target for plant extracts: Inhibition of bacterial quorum sensing. Journal of Molecular Biology and Biotechnology. 2016;**1**(1)1-3

[59] Lee NK, Paik HD. Status, antimicrobial mechanism, and regulation of natural preservatives in livestock food systems. Korean Journal for Food Science of Animal Resources. 2016;**36**(4):547-557

[60] Dizaj SM, Lotfipour F, Barzegar-Jalali M, Zarrintan MH, Adibkia K. Antimicrobial activity of the metals and metal oxide nanoparticles. Materials Science and Engineering: C. 2014;**44**:278-284

[61] Abdallah EM. Plants: An alternative source for antimicrobials. Journal of Applied Pharmaceutical Science. 2011;**1**(6):16-20

[62] Veerapandian M, Yun K. Functionalization of biomolecules on nanoparticles: Specialized for antibacterial applications. Applied Microbiology and Biotechnology. 2011;**90**(5): 1655-1667

Chapter 4

Silver Nanoparticles as Multi-Functional Drug Delivery Systems

Nadezhda Ivanova, Viliana Gugleva,
Mirena Dobreva, Ivaylo Pehlivanov,
Stefan Stefanov and Velichka Andonova

Additional information is available at the end of the chapter

http://dx.doi.org/10.5772/intechopen.80238

Abstract

Nanoparticles can surmount some essential problems of conventional small molecules or biomacromolecules (e.g., DNA, RNA, and protein) used in some diseases by allowing targeted delivery and overcome through biological barriers. Recently, silver nanoparticles have been harnessed as delivery vehicles for therapeutic agents, including antisense oligonucleotides, and other small molecules. Silver is the most profit-oriented precious metal used in the preparation of nanoparticles and nanomaterials because of its antibacterial, antiviral, antifungal, antioxidant and unusually enhanced physicochemical properties compared to the bulk material such as optical, thermal, electrical, and catalytic properties. Small silver nanoparticles offer many advantages as drug carriers, including adjustable size and shape, enhanced stability of surface-bound nucleic acids, high-density surface ligand attachment, transmembrane delivery without harsh transfection agents, protection of the attached therapeutics from degradation, and potential for improved timed/controlled intracellular drug-delivery. Plant-mediated synthesis of silver nanoparticles is gaining interest due to its inexpensiveness, providing a healthier work environment, and protecting human health leading to lessening waste and safer products. The chapter presents the essential physicochemical characteristics, antibacterial, and anticancer properties which silver nanoparticles obtained by plant-mediated methods possess, and their application as drug-delivery systems with a critical view on the possible toxicity on the human body.

Keywords: antibacterial activity, anticancer activity, capping agents, plant extracts, reducing agents, surface properties, toxicity

1. Introduction

Nanomedicine is a branch of medicine that uses nanomaterials and applies nanotechnologies in prevention, diagnostics, and treatment of diseases [1]. The broad definition of nanomedicine involves nanoparticles (NPs) as drug delivery systems (DDSs), medical nanosensor, biochips, insulin pumps, needleless injectors, etc. The unique properties of NPs are related to their tiny size (generally between 1 and 100 nm), huge surface area, and surface characteristics. "Nano" DDSs provide targeted delivery of optimal dose with reduced side effects and toxicity. Moreover, NPs solve problems related to drug solubility and bioavailability. These "nano" carriers can protect the drug from the hazardous environment as well as to overcome the biological barriers to entry the drug to the targeted tissues and to deal with drug resistance. They possess organic or inorganic origin and can be prepared from different polymers, metals, ceramics, etc.

Silver is the most profit-oriented precious metal used in the preparation of NPs and nanomaterials. These are known because their antibacterial, antiviral, antifungal, antioxidant, and unusually enhanced physicochemical properties compared to the bulk material such as optical, thermal, electrical, and catalytic properties [2–5]. About 500 tons of silver nanoparticles (AgNPs), used in various industries and everyday life, are produced per year [6, 7]. Rising demand for silver nanomaterials requires the development of eco-friendly synthesis methods. In general, AgNPs can be produced by chemical, physical, and biological methods. Chemical protocols are mainly based on the chemical reduction of Ag+ ions by organic and inorganic agents, such as sodium borohydride, sodium citrate, sodium ascorbate, elemental hydrogen, N, N-dimethylformamide, polymers, Tollens methods, etc. The reducing agent reduces Ag^+ and leads to the formation of Ag^0, metallic silver, which agglomerates into oligomeric clusters. These clusters may form colloidal particles of metallic silver. Different surfactants and polymers are used to prevent particles from further agglomeration and protect their shape [8]. The most important physical methods are based on evaporation-condensation technique and laser ablation of silver bulk material in solution. Both physical approaches did not use chemical reagents that may be hazardous to the environment and the human body. Although these require costly specialized equipment, physical methods provide an alternative to environmentally unfriendly and time-consuming chemical protocols.

Biological or so-called "green" methods do not use toxic chemicals in the preparation techniques. Moreover, these methods are based on the usage of bacteria, fungi, algae, and plants to obtain AgNPs characterized by size and shape depending optical, electrical, and antimicrobial properties [8, 9]. These are based on bioreduction of Ag+ ions in the aqueous medium where the reducing agents are cited above biological sources. Synthesis of AgNPs using living microorganisms (bacteria and fungi) can be performed either intracellularly or extracellularly [10]. The extracellular synthesis is cheaper, less time-consuming, and requires simplified manufacturing technology compared to the intracellular synthesis. Studies used culture supernatants of pathogenic and nonpathogenic microorganisms like *A. flavus*, *B. indicus*, *B. cereus*, *Bacillus* strain CS 11, *E. coli*, *P. proteolytica*, *P. meridiana*, *S. aureus*, etc. [10–12]. The drawbacks of bacterial synthesis of AgNPs are related to the selection and cultivation of suitable bacterial strain, a mandatory stage of purification, the poor understanding of the mechanisms governing the nanoparticle formation which hinders scaling laboratory process in the industry as well as the requirements of highly aseptic conditions and their maintenance [13].

Plant-mediated green synthesis of AgNPs is gaining immense popularity because of its eco-friendly nature, accessibility, economy, execution-simplicity, and the possibility of large-scale production. Many studies have used different plant extracts such as *Azadirachta indica*, *Crocus sativus* L., *Calliandra haematocephala*, Neem leaves, *Madhuca longifolia*, grape seed extract, *Andean blackberry* fruit extract, geranium leaf aqueous extract, marigold flower, etc. [7, 14–19]. The rich phytochemical composition of the extracts used implies its complex action, for example, as reducing, stabilizing, and capping agents. The AgNPs thus obtained can be exploited as DDSs for different active pharmaceutical ingredients.

The chapter presents the essential physicochemical characteristics, antibacterial, and anticancer properties, which AgNPs obtained by plant-mediated methods possess, and their application as DDSs with a critical view on the possible toxicity on the human body.

2. Plant-mediated synthesis of silver nanoparticles

It is well known that plant extracts have a rich phytochemical composition including phenolics, saponins, terpenoids, flavonoids, catechins, tannins, enzymes, proteins, polysaccharides, etc. All of these biomolecules take place in a very complicated mechanism of reduction and stabilization of Ag+ ions to form AgNPs. For example, Li et al. suggested a recognition-reduction-limited nucleation and growth model to explain the possible formation mechanism of AgNPs in *Capsicum annuum* L. extract [19]. According to the authors, the proteins which have amine groups played a reducing and controlling role during the formation of AgNPs in the solutions, and that the secondary structure of the proteins changed after reaction with Ag+ ions. In another study, Mirgorod and Borodina, based on the surface-enhanced Raman spectroscopy data, stated that the NPs were formed as a result of a redox reaction between flavonoids and Ag+ ions as well as there are flavonoids near the surface of the AgNPs, which react complexly with Ag+ ions and with the NPs [20]. Ahmed and co-workers described different approaches of syntheses of AgNPs and protocols employed for their synthesis in detail [21].

It is important to note that technological parameters such as temperature, pH, the concentration of Ag+ ions, duration of the obtaining process, phytochemical composition of the extract used, mechanical stirring, microwave assistance, etc., are crucial both for nanoparticle preparation and for their characteristics and fate [6, 7, 14–19]. These parameters affect not only the process of reduction of Ag+ ion and formation of metallic silver but also its agglomeration into oligomeric clusters which may form colloidal particles with specific features. Amin and co-workers found that the time of reaction, temperature, and volume ratio of methanol extract from *Solanum xanthocarpum* berry to $AgNO_3$ could accelerate the reduction rate of Ag+ ions and affect the AgNPs size and shape [22]. The NPs were found to be about 10 nm in size, mono-dispersed in nature, and spherical in shape.

Surface functionality of nanomaterials is crucial for their applicability, compatibility, and safety. Generally, surface behavior defines how a nano-entity will interact with biosystems, environment, etc. [23]. AgNPs are characterized with variable morphology—size, shape, surface area, purity/coating—and related electrochemical and electromagnetic properties—charge, zeta potential, redox potential, surface plasmon resonance, and conductivity [24, 25]. A change or intentional attempt to control these essential characteristics is an essential tool in tailoring AgNPs for specific purposes and might be highly sought on several accounts: (1) increased stability; (2) increased selectivity; (3) increased therapeutic or diagnostic potency; (4) enhanced catalytic activity; (5) reduced toxicity; and (6) reduced reactivity [23, 25]. Surface functionalization of AgNPs may be determined by the synthesis pathway chosen (one-step functionalization) or additional treatment after isolation (multi-step functionalization).

3. Surface properties of silver nanoparticles

3.1. Purity on the surface of "green" synthesized AgNPs

The "green" synthesis of AgNPs using plant extracts often results not only in deliberate, but also inevitable surface functionalization because every component in the total aqueous plant extract (being reducers, stabilizers, or concomitant constituents) has a certain affinity to the silver surface [16, 24, 26]. After isolation and purification, surface remain only those components which can bind the strongest is "attached" to the AgNPs. Sorption, or so-called "attachment," might occur due to chemical (chemisorption) or physical (physisorption) phenomenon. Chemisorption, in the case of AgNPs, happens via ionic, covalent, or coordinate-covalent chemical bonds. S-containing molecules (some amino acids, peptides, and proteins) possess the highest affinity to the silver surface because of the strong Ag-S bond and hence are the first to be considered for interaction [17, 26–28]. Next, N and O atoms from amide, amino, hydroxyl, phenol, carboxyl, and carbonyl groups are targets for complex formation with Ag^+ ions and thus also very likely to be absorbed on the surface [7, 15, 16, 18, 25–30]. The latter exist in most primary and secondary metabolites in plants (phenolic acids, polyphenols, flavanoids alkaloids, glycosides, polysaccharides proteins, etc.) and are found to be present on AgNPs' surface by many researchers [7, 15–18, 24, 28, 31]. Physisorption arises due to Van der Waals forces, and though is much weaker compared to chemisorption; it is non-specific and can affect every polarized unit in the AgNP's surrounding. Knowing that the electric potential of colloidal silver can be considerable, this explains the significant role of physisorption for the surface functionalization of "green" synthesized AgNPs. It has to be noted, that regardless the mechanism, biomolecules participating in Ag^+ ion reduction, are more likely to enter in an interaction with the silver surface because of their initial intimate contact with the arising particles [7, 15–18, 24, 31].

A question may arise whether this heterogenic and uncontrollable "impurity" on AgNPs' surface following "green" synthesis with plant extracts is only advantageous or does it have any weak sides. In fact, this highly depends on the particles' designation. The presence of tannins, proteins, polysaccharides, flavonoids, and lipids has been proven to benefit stability, increases

AgNPs' catalytic, antibacterial, and antioxidant activity and reduces toxicity by passivation of the surface [7, 14–16, 21, 31–34]. However, the "coating" of AgNPs reduces their size and agglomeration rate, as well as some researchers, suggest that this may have an adverse effect on cytotoxicity [33]. Furthermore, for surface-selective analytical techniques (such as surface-enhanced Raman spectroscopy, SERS), where the use of AgNPs provides promising results as enhancers, a "clear" surface is required that allows access to targeted analytes [26]. In this regard, the use of pure natural reducers (e.g., the flavonoids quercetin, chrysin, apigenin, luteolin, etc.) might be preferable instead of the total plant extract [25, 26, 28, 35]. However, if the presence of multicomponent and unpredictable adherence on the AgNPs is unwelcome, still the need for a "capping" agent exists. Sugars and polysaccharides, proteins and proteoglycans as glucose, galactose, mannose, chitosan, sodium alginate, glucans, gelatin, and others are commonly used as coatings for the purpose [17, 27, 35, 36]. These are most often being included in the reduction media during synthesis, whereas the mechanisms of their attachment to the surface follow the above-described principles [27, 35].

3.2. The surface area of AgNPs

The active surface area of AgNPs is determined by their size, shape, and agglomeration rate. Reaction conditions as pH, temperature, extract volume and concentration, reactants ratio, and time define the dimensions and degree of crystal growth and thus affect the size and shape of the silver aggregates [16, 24, 25, 31].

The polydispersity of the resulting AgNPs is a disadvantage of the "green" synthesis with plant extracts, which is likely due to the uncontrollable deposition of different compounds on the surface and the heterogeneity of the reaction media. In this regard, the use of an o/w microemulsion-upgraded method has shown good results [18]. Post-synthesis agglomeration may lead to enlargement of the aggregates and eventually to colloid instability. Here is the role of the "cap" on AgNPs' surface, which is aimed to overcome the attractive forces between the particles and increase physical stability. A large surface area is desirable because it provides greater catalytic and antibacterial efficacy due to the increased $Ag+$ release from the surface which is a fundamental mechanism of AgNPs' antibacterial action [25, 32]. However, this precise mechanism, proven by many, is also related to increased oxidative stress and cytotoxicity [33, 35]. Furthermore, AgNPs smaller than 10 nm can pass through the nuclear pores and interact with chromosomes and DNA. Thus such particles are proper for gene therapy and diagnostics, but dangerous regarding genotoxicity [33]. On the one hand, each intervention leading to suppression of particles' agglomeration and reducing their size is welcome concerning stability and potency in catalysis, antibacterial therapy, and diagnostics. On the other hand, the same intervention can be potentially hazardous concerning increased toxicity of the NPs obtained [25, 33, 35].

The shape of AgNPs has also been demonstrated to have an impact on toxicity [34, 37]. For example, wire-shaped AgNPs have shown higher toxicity compared to spherical NPs [37], whereas another study testifies that plate-shaped AgNPs' toxic potential exceeds those of wires and spheres [34].

3.3. Electrochemical and electromagnetic properties of AgNPs

The charge and zeta potential of AgNPs occurring in suspension are main factors determining the stability of the colloidal system and depend highly on the synthesis of variables as well. Among them, pH of the reaction media and the type of coating are crucial [31, 35]. Zeta potential (ζ) is the potential occurring between the surface of AgNPs and the surrounding liquid phase and is an important measure for the stability of colloidal systems. Values beyond $\zeta = \pm 30$ mV are usually taken as a requirement for colloid's endurance [31]. Adjustment of pH during synthesis is considered an electrostatic approach for stabilization of colloids (by changing the type and quantity of the electric charge), whereas the coating aims to diminish the attractive forces in a steric way [31, 35]. AgNPs obtained by reduction with plant extracts most often are negatively charged [7, 15, 17, 18, 27, 29, 35]. The negative zeta potential can be considered an advantage because increased cellular uptake and subsequent cytotoxicity are found for positively charged AgNPs [23, 33].

The presence of "capping" agents on the surface is essential for the stability of colloidal systems, but they also affect the so-called "redox potential" of AgNPs, that is, their ability to acquire electrons and be reduced [38]. Low redox potential is needed for oxidation on the surface and Ag^+ release and therefore promotes higher antibacterial activity and toxicity [33]. In some cases, the immobilization of AgNPs in slightly permeable "cap" may lead to loss of ability for oxidation and antibacterial properties [35].

The surface plasmon resonance (SPR) is a characteristic optical property of AgNPs due to resonant oscillation of electrons on the surface caused by irradiation with light [39]. This electromagnetic phenomenon results in an intense peak in the violet-blue sector of the visible spectrum [7, 15, 18, 24, 26]. The latter depends strongly on surface functionality (size, coating, etc.) and is considered proof for successful AgNPs synthesis [7, 15, 18, 24, 26, 39].

3.4. Association of AgNPs in complexes and delivery vehicles

A few attempts to incorporate "green" synthesized AgNPs in the structure of liposomes, cyclodextrins, nanoemulsions, and hydrogel beads are reported. Such approaches give the opportunity for targeted delivery, better compatibility, and lower toxicity [35, 40]. For example, one-step synthesis of AgNPs-stabilized liposomes have shown improved stability, compatibility, and antibacterial properties of resulting vesicles compared to AgNPs alone, also giving the opportunity for dermal delivery [40]. Other studies report that association of AgNPs with β-cyclodextrin improves their catalytic activity [25], whereas kappa-carrageenan hydrogel beads of "green" synthesized AgNPs have been found to deliver Ag^+ in a desirable controlled manner [41].

3.5. Functionalization by conjugation

Next level surface functionalization is the conjugation of AgNPs with bioactive molecules. This approach, unlike all of the above mentioned, can not only change but also lead to entirely new functions. The conjugation of oligonucleotides to metal nanoparticles' surface is widely researched for targeted gene therapy and bio-diagnostics. However, the attachment of DNA sequences on AgNPs surface has been challenging due to the lower stability of the complex. Few successful reports are available from the past years with disulfide or sulfhydryl inserted DNA [42, 43].

An exciting field of study is the AgNPs potential as drug-delivery carriers [29, 30, 44]. Hypotheses suggest that AgNPs can be used as vehicles to transport drug molecules to target zones and thereby improve therapeutical efficacy; furthermore, express synergism with synthetic antibiotics regarding antibacterial properties. These assumptions have been tested by several scientist in the field, who report successful conjugation of tetracycline (multiple hydroxyl, phenol, and amide groups), glycopeptide antibiotic vancomycin (multiple amide, phenol, and hydroxyl groups), and the immunosuppressant azathioprine (S-atom and basic N-atoms in heterocycle) [29, 30, 44].

4. Antibacterial activity of silver nanoparticles

Since ancient times elemental silver and its compounds have been used as antimicrobial agents. AgNPs synthesized by different methods were widely tested and had been proved effective against over 650 microorganisms including bacteria (both Gram-positive and Gram-negative), fungi, and viruses [21, 45]. Multiple mechanisms of antibacterial action of AgNPs are considered, but most studies simplified to three primary mechanisms: (1) adhesion of AgNPs onto the surface of cell wall and membrane; (2) penetration of AgNPs inside the cell and damaging of intracellular structures (mitochondria, vacuoles, and ribosomes), and biomolecules (protein, lipids, and DNA); and (3) generation of reactive oxygen species (ROS), leading to induced cellular toxicity, and oxidative stress [21, 45, 46]. According to Prabhu et al. and Dakal et al., modulation of signal transduction pathways is also a distinct mechanism of antimicrobial action of AgNPs [45, 47].

The adhesion of AgNPs onto the surface of the cell wall is facilitated by the positive surface charge of the AgNPs, and the occurred electrostatic attraction between AgNPs and the negatively charged cell membrane of microorganisms [48]. The interaction of Ag^{+} ions with the proteins containing sulfur, presented in the bacteria cell wall, irreversibly disrupted the bacterial cell wall [49]. The damage of cell membranes by AgNPs causing structural changes renders bacteria more permeable and disturbs the respiratory function [45, 46]. Morones et al. demonstrated the existence of silver in the membranes of treated bacteria as well as in the interior of it by transmission electron microscopy (TEM) analysis [50]. The composition and thickness of the cell wall also influence the antimicrobial potential of AgNPs [45, 48]. In Gram-negative bacteria such as *E. coli, Pseudomonas, Salmonella*, the cell wall consists of a layer of lipopolysaccharide, followed by a thin layer of peptidoglycan (3–4 nm). The cell wall in Gram-positive bacteria such as *Staphylococcus, Streptococcus, Bacillus* is mainly composed of a thick layer of peptidoglycan (30 nm thickness) [48, 51]. Hence, AgNPs exhibit greater antimicrobial effect against Gram-negative bacteria regardless of their resistance level as compared to Gram-positive bacteria [49].

It has also been proposed that Ag+ ion enters the cell and interacts with the sulfur and phosphorus of the DNA, which can lead to problems in the DNA replication of the bacteria and cell death [47].

The antibacterial potential of AgNPs has related also with the generation of free radicals and ROS and consequent increase in oxidative stress in cells. Silver ion can interact with the thiol groups of many vital enzymes, inactivate them and generate ROS. An excessive amount of generated free radicals lead to direct damage to mitochondrial membrane causing necrosis and eventually cell death [52].

The antimicrobial effect of AgNPs depends on various parameters including discussed above size, shape, zeta potential, dose, and colloidal state [15, 46, 49]. AgNPs having a size in the range of 10–100 nm showed strong bactericidal potential against both Gram-positive and Gram-negative bacteria [50, 51]. Depending on the size of the NPs, the large surface area comes in contact with the bacterial cells to provide a higher percentage of interaction than bigger particles [51, 53].

The effect of shape on the antibacterial activity of AgNPs has been studied by Pal et al. [54]. The AgNPs of different shapes (triangular, spherical, and rod) were tested against *E. coli*. According to the authors, triangular NPs are more active than spherical NPs, which are again more active than rod-shaped AgNPs against *E. coli*. This could be due to their larger surface area to volume ratios and their crystallographic surface structures [54]. Rout et al. synthesize AgNPs of different shapes (i.e., spherical, triangular, and rod) by using Mulberry (*Morus rubra L.*) leaves extract and studied their antibacterial activities against *E. coli* in both liquid systems and on an agar plate. High reactivity of the truncated triangular NPs has also been observed in comparison to spherical and rod-shaped particles [55].

Sondi and Salopeck-Sondi investigated the antibacterial activities of AgNPs against *E. coli* on Luria-Bertani agar plates and reported that the antibacterial activity of AgNPs was dose-dependent [56]. AgNPs in colloidal form, that is, suspended nano-sized Ag particles have shown enhanced antimicrobial potential over AgNPs alone. Colloidal AgNPs produced by green synthesis are characterized with controlled size, high stability, and improved antibacterial activity which is examined in different studies by directly exposing bacteria to AgNPs [45, 57].

Okafor et al. produced AgNPs by green synthesis from aloe, geranium, magnolia, and black cohosh extracts and studied their antibacterial activity on different species of bacteria: three Gram-negative and three Gram-positive bacteria [58]. The overall results indicated that the AgNPs showed antibacterial activity at doses of 2 and 4 ppm towards the Gram-positive and Gram-negative test bacteria. Aloe extract NPs showed the highest antibacterial activity, followed by black cohosh and geranium NPs with the lowest inhibition. The high antimicrobial effect of the aloe produced AgNPs may be due to a combination of the AgNPs and the aloe bioactive molecules (quinines and other aromatic compounds), which in combination enhanced the inactivation or growth inhibition of the bacteria species. In another study, Zhang and co-workers also reported that aloe-produced NPs have a high inhibitory growth in *E. coli* at low concentrations [59].

Ahmed et al. synthesized AgNPs using *Azadirachta indica* aqueous leaf extract and studied their antibacterial activity towards both Gram-positive (*S. aureus)* and Gram-negative (*E. coli*) bacterial strains compared with control and plant extract alone [7]. According to the authors, AgNPs showed effective antimicrobial properties compared to others due to their vast surface area providing better contact with the cell wall of microorganisms. Also, Bagherzade et al. synthesized AgNPs using an extract of saffron (*Crocus sativus* L.) [14]. The biosynthesized AgNPs showed a significant antibacterial effect against *E. coli, P. aeruginosa, K. pneumonia, S. flexneri,* and *B. subtilis.*

Gomathi et al. obtained spherical shaped AgNPs using *Datura stramonium* leaf extract and studied their antibacterial activity against *E. coli* and *S. aureus* using well diffusion technique [32]. The authors reported that AgNPs exhibited greater antibacterial activity against *E. coli* than *S. aureus,* due to the variation in cell wall membrane of these bacteria. In another study, spherical-shaped AgNPs with dimensions of 50–100 nm were observed using *Alternanthera dentate* aqueous extract and were tested against *E. coli, P. aeruginosa, K. pneumonia,* and *E. faecalis* by agar diffusion method [60]. The authors reported that the antibacterial effect of AgNPs was size- and dose-dependent and was more pronounced against Gram-negative bacteria than Gram-positive bacteria.

Antimicrobial activity of AgNPs with various antibiotics has been studied, and the synergistic antibacterial effect has been found. The bactericidal potential of AgNPs synthesized from the leaf extract of *Murraya koenigii* singly and in combination with antibiotics (gentamycin, ampicillin, and streptomycin) against the pathogenic bacteria, namely *E. coli, S. aureus,* and *P. aeruginosa* was studied [61]. The authors reported that AgNPs in combination with gentamycin showed the maximum activity against *E. coli* with an increase in fold area 4.06, while tetracycline combination with NPs showed maximum activity against *S. aureus.* The authors concluded that the activity of standard antibiotics was significantly increased in the presence of AgNPs and that can be used against antibiotic-resistant pathogens effectively.

5. Silver nanoparticles as anticancer drug delivery systems

Over the past years, nanomedicine created new horizon in the future development of anticancer strategies. Conventional cancer treatment such as chemotherapy, radiotherapy, or surgery has its limitations associated with drugs toxicity, unpredictable side effects, drug resistance problems, and lack of specificity. AgNPs overcome these disadvantages by reducing side effects and enhancing the efficiency of cancer therapy. One of their distinguishing features is the ability to cross various biological barriers and to provide targeted delivery of drugs. Green synthesis of AgNPs together with specific delivery of anticancer drugs to tumor tissues offers an innovative approach for improving cancer treatment [62].

5.1. Anticancer activity of biologically synthesized AgNPs

The anticancer activity of biologically synthesized AgNPs has been studied using both *in vitro* and *in vivo* models. The reported results suggested that cytotoxicity of AgNPs may be influenced by particle size, shape, and surface chemistry. Several authors have claimed that increasing AgNPs concentration the viability of tumor cells decreases [63, 64].

The effect of time and concentration of AgNPs on inhibition of cell viability and membrane leakage are evaluated with a variety of methods [65, 66]. Usually, MTT assay, quantification of ROS, RT-PCR, and western blotting techniques are used for the assessment of AgNPs ability to inhibit cellular growth and mediate cell death [65–68]. *In vitro* cytotoxic activity in a dose-dependent manner was estimated for green synthesized AgNPs from different plants—*Vitex negundro* L., *Acalypha indica, Euphorbia nivulia,* and *Premna serratifolia* [63]. *MCF-7* (human breast adenocarcinoma) cell lines were treated with AgNPs obtained by the use of *Erythrina indica* and *Andrographis echioides* extracts. In both cases, the growth of cancer cells was inhibited following AgNPs concentration-response relationship [63]. Similar results were found in other studies [65, 67]. The AgNPs obtained by use of *Artemisia marshalliana* Sprengel extract and *Ganoderma neo-japonicum* Imazeki extract had a confirmed cytotoxic potential on human gastric cancer *AGS* cell line and *MDA-MB-231* human breast cancer cell. The authors found that the cytotoxic activity of AgNPs was time- and dose-dependent as well as the size of NPs and the temperature of the preparation process.

Dependence on anticancer activity of AgNPs on human cancer cell lines has been found, according to the source for the synthesis of NPs as well as on the type of the cell lines [69]. Extracts from fruits, leaves, seeds, and roots of *Citrullus colocynthis* produced AgNPs with different size and alteration in ID_{50} on various cell lines. The toxicity assay of biologically synthesized AgNPs using seaweed *Ulva lactuca* showed potential cytotoxicity of AgNPs against tumors. For human colon cancer, *HT-29* cell lines ID_{50} was 49 μg/ml whereas its value reached 12.5 μg/ml in human liver cancer *Hep G-2* cell lines.

One of the significant drawbacks of conventional anticancer therapy is drug-mediated toxicity in healthy cells. AgNPs synthesized from plants have the potential to avoid this problem by offering selective toxicity to cancer cells. AgNPs produced using leaf extract of *Podophyllum hexandrum* Royle induced cytotoxicity to cervical carcinoma cells. The reported results proved that AgNPs could selectively inhibit the cellular mechanism of *HeLa* by DNA damage and caspase-mediated cell death [70]. In another study, the cytotoxicity of AgNPs towards cancer cells was estimated comparing human myeloblastic leukemia cells *HL60* and cervical cancer cells *HeLa* to normal peripheral blood mononuclear cells (*PBMC*) [66]. *Sargassum vulgare* had been used for the green synthesis of AgNPs. It was found that *HL60* cells were affected by AgNP-mediated toxicity while the normal *PBMC* suffered less damage.

It has been proven that biologically synthesized AgNPs show substantial anticancer activity with less toxic manner compared to particles whose preparation involves some toxic and expensive chemicals. The production AgNPs through green chemistry approach via *Cleome viscosa* plant extract offers another solution for optimizing anticancer treatment. Anticancer activity was *in vitro* evaluated against human cancer cell lines *PA1* (Ovarian teratocarcinoma cell line) and *A549* (Human lung adenocarcinoma) [68]. The results concluded that green synthesized AgNPs could inhibit cancer cells growth and provide great potential in the treatment of cancer.

To determine the anticancer efficacy of biologically synthesized AgNPs and to fully apprehend the mode of programmed cell death three critical parameters need to be taken into consideration: (1) DNA fragmentation; (2) structural changes in the cell morphology; and (3) Annexin V binding and caspase activation. Upregulation of apoptosis is only one of the possible mechanisms for antiproliferative activity of biosynthesized AgNPs that was proven in many studies [67, 71, 72]. AgNPs could elicit cell death through ROS generation, membrane leakage, activation of caspases, and DNA damage [65, 66, 72].

5.2. AgNPs for targeted drug delivery

AgNPs represent an alternative therapeutic strategy as DDSs in curing cancer because these can provide passive or active targeting to tumor tissue. Accumulation of drugs at desired sites increases the efficacy of anticancer therapy *in vivo*. Receptor-mediated endocytosis can facilitate cellular uptake of drugs. This kind of active targeting relays on molecular recognition. Suggested approach for optimizing biogenic AgNPs properties is surface functionalization with specific targeting molecules or coating with biocompatible and biodegradable polymers [73, 74]. For example, AgNPs obtained by use of various concentrations of *Setaria verticillata* seed extract were loaded with hydrophilic anticancer drugs, doxorubicin (DOX), and daunorubicin (DNR). The significant loading (80.50%) and capacity (40.25%) efficiency of DOX-AgNPs and DNR-AgNPs presented them as future novel DDSs [64].

Drug delivery into the cells by endocytosis depends on the size of NPs. Spherical-shaped AgNPs were extracted from *Aerva javanica* plant and conjugated with the anti-cancer drug gefitinib. Scanning transmission electron microscopy (STEM) images determinates average size of 5.7 nm. The apoptotic potential of gefitinib-AgNPs has been compared to gefitinib alone. Reduction of cell viability of breast cancer cells *MCF-7* treated with conjugated gefitinib-AgNPs was significant. Delivery of gefitinib using AgNPs optimizes its effectivity and reduces side effects [75].

The variety of green synthesized AgNPs exhibiting anticancer activity offer new treatment opportunities. Their specific features as nanocarriers benefit the development of DDSs with unique properties and biocompatible profile.

6. Silver nanoparticles as photoactivated drug delivery vectors

Nanoparticles can surmount some essential problems of conventional small molecules or biomacromolecules (e.g., DNA, RNA, and protein) used at some diseases by allowing targeted delivery and overcome through biological barriers [76]. Noble metal NPs have specific high developed photophysical properties which contribute to their potential as photoactivated drug delivery vectors [77]. AgNPs have been used extensively as biological sensors which take advantage of plasmon resonance (PR) to enhance detection of specific targets. Noble metal nanoparticle-based sensors benefit from the extreme sensitivity of localized surface plasmon resonance (LSPR) spectra to environmental changes. Application of metal nanoparticles is not limited to molecular detection. Recently, AgNPs have been harnessed as delivery vehicles for therapeutic agents, including antisense oligonucleotides and other small molecules. Small metal NPs offer many advantages as drug carriers, including adjustable size and shape, enhanced stability of surface-bound nucleic acids, high-density surface ligand attachment, transmembrane delivery without harsh transfection agents, protection of the attached therapeutic from degradation, and potential for improved timed/controlled intracellular release. The photophysical properties of AgNPs may potentially bring these to the forefront of drug delivery, enabling targeted delivery, spatiotemporally controlled (photo-)release, and delivery confirmation via imaging [78].

AgNPs in the diameter range of ~2–100 nm exhibit SPR spectra in the visible region, which are tunable and dependent on particle shape, size, environment, and interparticle distance. AgNPs have unique properties which make them a desirable alternative particle type in many cases. AgNPs are the strongest light scatterers of the noble metal particles, and it is reported that the light scattering cross section of AgNP is ~10 times greater than that of a similarly sized gold NPs. The extinction (light absorption and scattering) band of AgNPs is due to free conduction electron oscillations, and bound electron movements also contribute to the optical spectra. Thus enhancement of absorption/emission of light by molecules near the AgNPs surface is dependent on particle size and proximity or overlap of the resonance (SPR) spectra with the absorption/emission bands of the molecular species [78].

Mie Theory has calculated the light absorption and scattering properties for AgNPs of different sizes. For larger particle sizes (~50–60 nm), the scattering efficiency (Qsca) is higher (≈ 5). The AgNPs in this size range scatter light at or above the solid metal surface, but the scattering efficiency increases even higher to 5.8 for size 70–80 nm while maintaining surface PR in the UV to the visible range. This characteristic is ideal for traditional and red-shifted photocleavable compounds typically used as photo-caging compounds [78].

The generality of current nanoscale delivery systems are polymeric in their essence. The studies of metallic NPs have shown their suitability for delivery of various therapeutic agents including small molecules, antisense oligonucleotides, and siRNAs. Nanoscale silver is one of the optically active surface-enhancing substrates available. AgNP-based single delivery platforms incorporate solutions to both intracellular detection and external control over surface-tethered drug release via chemical photothermal or photochemical triggers [77].

Light-responsive systems are of great interest in the field of drug delivery and gene therapy, owing to the capability of external, spatiotemporal control over the delivery, and activation of therapeutics coupled with such systems. Electromagnetic radiation triggers light-responsive DDSs, typically in the UV, visible, and near-infrared (NIR) range. These systems are based upon photosensitive compounds which can be incorporated into a drug delivery vehicle, or coupled to the drug itself ("caging" compounds), and may switch to an active or inactive state upon electromagnetic irradiation within a specific frequency range. Caged compounds are potent tools for spatiotemporal control over drug activity in living systems. Photocleavable groups have been used to the cage, or inactivate, various biomolecules, including nucleotides, proteins, and nucleic acids, for controlled, on-site photo-activation. Uncaging via light irradiation allows rapid, spatially, and temporally defined release of a biomolecule at intended tissues or even within a specific intracellular compartment [78].

AgNPs with the size of 60–80 nm decorated with thiol-terminated photolabile DNA oligonucleotides were used as photo-activated drug delivery vectors [77]. *In vitro* assays showed efficient photo-activation of surface-tethered caged ISIS2302 antisense oligonucleotides with internal photo-cleavable linkers. These nanocarriers have several advantages such as protection against nucleases, efficient photorelease, and enhanced cellular uptake when compared to commercial transfection agents. The light-induced release of anti-sense oligonucleotides for silencing ICAM-1 (intracellular adhesion molecule-1) has potential application in the wound healing, where inflammation is a significant criterion such as in Crohn's disease.

7. Toxicity assessment of silver nanoparticles

Nanotechnology has been rapidly growing with utilization in a wide range of commercial products throughout the world. However, there is still a lack of information concerning the increase of human, animal, and environmental exposure to NPs including AgNPs and the potential risks related to their short- and long-term toxicity. However, some studies have already been made.

7.1. *In vitro* tests

AgNPs have emerged as an important class of nanomaterials for a wide range of industrial and medical applications that have potential risks to human health. *In vitro* studies reported, that AgNPs produced toxicity targeted a variety of organs including the lung, liver, brain, vascular system, and reproductive organs. AgNPs induced the expression level of genes involved in cell cycle progression and apoptosis. Possible mechanisms of AgNP toxicity include induction of ROS, oxidative stress, DNA damage, and apoptosis [79].

To understand the toxicity of NPs *in vitro* different tests have been assessed. Testing silver (Ag – 15 nm), molybdenum (MoO_3–30 nm), and aluminum (Al – 30 nm) NPs on mouse spermatogonial cell line have been determined concentration-dependent toxicity for all types. AgNPs were the most toxic (5–10 μg ml^{-1}), and reduced mitochondrial function drastically and increased membrane leakage [80]. Similar conclusions have been made testing the toxic effects of the metal/metal oxides NPs mentioned above on rat liver-derived cell line (*BRL 3A*). Results showed that mitochondrial function decreases significantly in cells exposed to AgNPs at (5–50 μg ml^{-1}). Fe_3O_4, Al, MoO_3, and TiO_2 had no measurable effect at lower doses (10–50 μg ml^{-1}), while there was a significant effect at higher levels (100–250 μg ml^{-1}) [81].

Generally, in *in vitro* tests, the mechanism of AgNPs-mediated cytotoxicity is mainly based on the induction of ROS. Notably, exposure to AgNPs causes a reduction in GSH, elevated ROS levels, lipid peroxidation, and increased expression of ROS responsive genes; it also leads to DNA damage, apoptosis, and necrosis. MTT (3-(4,5-dimethylthiazol-2-yl)-2,5-diphenyl tetrazolium bromide) reduction, Alamar Blue (Invitrogen, Carlsbad, CA) reduction, and lactate dehydrogenase (LDH) leakage were used as parameters for cytotoxicity assessment. Toxicity of different AgNPs was compared to that of various corresponding concentrations of Ag+ ions. Based upon the IC50 values determined by three cytotoxicity assays, AgNPs and Ag+ ions did not exhibit a dramatic difference in cytotoxicity [82]. The cytotoxicity and genotoxicity of AgNPs are size-, concentration-, and exposure time-dependent. The cell viability was determined by MTT and CB assay in macrophage (*RAW 264.7, J774.1*), pulmonary epithelial (*A549*), renal epithelial (*A498*), hepatic (*Hep G2*), and neuronal (*Neuro 2A*) cell lines. AgNPs showed a concentration-dependent reduction in cell viability after 72 h incubation in all cell lines. *A498* and *RAW 264.7* cells appeared to exhibit the highest sensitivity to the toxic effects of AgNPs and showed significant reduction in cell viability at 1 and 3 g/ml AgNP-concentration, respectively. On the other hand, *A549* cells were least sensitive to cytotoxic effects of AgNPs. The internalization of NPs can induce stress response(s) due to stimulation of free radical production, which in turn, stimulates inflammatory signaling pathways. Hence, the production of reactive nitrogen species (RNS), ROS, and cytokines following AgNPs exposure was determined. AgNPs significantly increased nitrite release by *RAW 264.7* cells at the highest concentration following 72 h incubation. AgNPs also stimulated ROS production in a concentration-dependent manner after 24 h incubation. Inflammatory cytokine (tumor necrosis factor-α [TNF-α] and interleukin-6 [IL-6]) production was significant at 10 and 100 g/ml while 1 g/ml showed no effect on cytokine production. Free radical production has been demonstrated to bear a direct correlation with cytotoxicity of NPs. However, the involvement of other mechanisms cannot be ruled out. Therefore, to determine the contribution of free radicals in AgNP cytotoxicity, cells were incubated with AgNPs in the presence of various antioxidants. Surprisingly, the most potent antioxidants like superoxide dismutase (SOD) and catalase showed no significant protection from AgNPs cytotoxicity. Therefore, two cell membrane ROS scavengers—Trolox (water-soluble vitamin E analog) and tempol (broad-spectrum antioxidant and SOD mimetic)—were investigated. In line with observations in SOD and catalase-treated cells, Trolox and tempol also failed to protect cells from AgNPs cytotoxicity. On the other hand, weak antioxidants like N-acetylcysteine (NAC), methionine and cysteine abrogated the cytotoxic effect of AgNPs. The relative ineffectiveness of potent antioxidants suggests that free radical-dependent mechanisms do not significantly influence cytotoxicity of AgNPs [83]. Other studies showed that p53 protein expression level increased within 4 h after the cells were exposed to AgNPs. The up-regulated expression patterns of p53 protein in two types of mammalian cells by AgNPs exposure suggest that the p53 could be an excellent molecule marker to assess the genetic nanotoxicity. The results suggest the different surface chemistry of AgNPs have different effects on genotoxicity [84]. Beer et al. concluded that free Ag+ ions in AgNPs preparations play a considerable role in the toxicity of AgNPs suspensions [85]. While the contribution of the free Ag+ ion to the measured toxicity of AgNPs suspensions is an essential determinant for the toxicity, a combined effect of Ag+ ion and AgNPs appears for lower concentrations of Ag+ ions. These data indicate that the amount of Ag+ ions in AgNPs preparations should be routinely measured and reported in toxicological work. They advise that the supernatant of AgNPs suspensions should be used as an additional standard control to make reliable statements of the toxicity of AgNPs and to discriminate between Ag+ ions toxicity and AgNPs-induced toxicity [85].

7.2. *In vivo* tests

The most significant problem to understand is the real impact of AgNPs on human health and animals. There are several *in vivo* studies on cytotoxicity and genotoxicity of AgNPs reported. Due to the ultra-small sizes of AgNPs, they have high mobility in different environments, and humans are easily exposed via routes such as inhalation, ingestion, skin, etc. AgNPs can translocate from the route of exposure to other vital organs and penetrate into cells.

Inhalation toxicity of AgNPs has been investigated on Sprague–Dawley rats over a period of 28 days. Results showed that the male and female rats did not show any significant changes in body weight relative to the concentration of AgNPs during the 28-day experiment. There were also no significant changes in the hematology and blood biochemical values in either the male or female rats. Whereas, some investigators have reported that lungs are primary target tissues affected by prolonged inhalation exposure to AgNPs [86]. Lee et al. have reported AgNPs exposure modulated the expression of several genes associated with motor neuron disorders, neurodegenerative disease, and immune cell function, indicating potential neurotoxicity and immunotoxicity associated with AgNPs exposure [87]. Minimal pulmonary inflammation or cytotoxicity of mice was found after 10 days of AgNPs exposure. Gastrointestinal toxicology caused by AgNPs (60 nm) exposure via ingestion has also been tested over a period of 28 days in Sprague–Dawley rats. Results showed that the male and female rats did not show any significant changes in body weight relative to the doses of AgNPs during the 28-day experiment. Some significant dose-dependent changes were found in the alkaline phosphatase and cholesterol values in either the male or female rats, seeming to indicate that exposure to over more than 300 mg of AgNPs may result in slight liver damage. Results suggested that AgNPs do not induce genetic toxicity in male and female rat bone marrow *in-vivo* [88]. Ahamed et al. indicated that AgNPs produce reproductive failure, developmental malformations, and morphological deformities in some non-mammalian animal models. Common causes of AgNPs-induced toxicity include oxidative stress, DNA damage, and apoptosis [79].

Generally, very few papers on the *in vivo* toxicology of AgNPs were found, so further investigation is needed in this field to evaluate precisely the real impact of AgNPs in commercial products to humans and animals.

8. Conclusion

Plant-mediated synthesis of AgNPs has revealed new horizons in drug-delivery. On the one hand, this approach of nanoparticle preparation is preferable due to its economic, accessible, eco-friendly nature, and simplicity of execution. On the other hand, the rich phytochemical composition of plant extracts performs a multi-functional role in the synthesis process of AgNPs as reducing, stabilizing, and the surface-active agent. The AgNPs thus obtained are usually characterized by tiny sizes, monodispersity, and stability of colloidal system because of the capping properties of some of the biomolecules in the extract. Despite their excellent antibacterial, antiviral, antifungal, anticancer, antioxidant, and unusually enhanced physicochemical properties compared to the bulk material, the AgNPs could be used as vehicles to transport drug molecules (such as oligonucleotides, DNA, siRNA, etc.) to targeted tissues and cells and thereby to improve therapeutic efficacy. Moreover, AgNPs could express synergism with different antibiotics regarding enhanced antibacterial properties. In this regard, the AgNPs might be used as multi-functional drug carriers having great potential in targeted drug-delivery, minimizing side effects, and improving therapeutic efficacy. However, there is still a lack of information concerning the increase of human, animal, and environmental exposure to AgNPs and the potential risks related to their short- and long-term toxicity. Further profound investigations are needed for their safe inclusion as DDSs in commercially available products for the prevention and treatment of life-threatening diseases.

Conflict of interest

The authors have declared no conflicts of interest for this article.

Author details

Nadezhda Ivanova, Viliana Gugleva, Mirena Dobreva, Ivaylo Pehlivanov, Stefan Stefanov and Velichka Andonova*

*Address all correspondence to: andonova_v@abv.bg

Department of Pharmaceutical Technologies, Faculty of Pharmacy, Medical University – Varna "Prof. Dr. Paraskev Stoyanov", Varna, Bulgaria

References

[1] Satalkar P, Elger BS, Shaw DM. Defining nano, nanotechnology and nanomedicine: Why should it matter? Science and Engineering Ethics. 2016;**22**(5):1255-1276

[2] Le Ouay B, Stellacci F. Antibacterial activity of silver nanoparticles: A surface science insight. Nano Today. 2015;**10**(3):339-354

[3] Phull A-R, Abbas Q, Ali A, Raza H, Kim SJ, Zia M, Haq I. Antioxidant, cytotoxic and antimicrobial activities of green synthesized silver nanoparticles from crude extract of *Bergenia ciliata*. FJPS. 2016;**2**(1):31-36

[4] Tolaymat TM, El Badawy AM, Genaidy A, Scheckel KG, Luxton TP, Suidan M. An evidence-based environmental perspective of manufactured silver nanoparticle in syntheses and applications: A systematic review and critical appraisal of peer-reviewed scientific papers. Science of the Total Environment. 2010;**408**(5):999-1006

[5] CD Creative diagnostics®. CD Bioparticles products. Properties and Application of Silver Nanoparticles. Available from: https://www.cd-bioparticles.com/t/Properties-and-Applications-of-Silver-Nanoparticles_60.html [Accessed: 2018-06-16]

[6] Larue C, Michel H, Sobanska S, Cécillon L, Bureau S, Barthès V, et al. Foliar exposure of the crop *Lactuca sativa* to silver nanoparticles: Evidence for internalization and changes in Ag speciation. Journal of Hazardous Materials. 2014;**264**:98-106

[7] Ahmed S, Saifullah, Ahmad M, Swami BL, Ikram S. Green synthesis of silver nanoparticles using *Azadirachta indica* aqueous leaf extract. Journal of Radiation Research and Applied Science. 2016;**9**:1-7

[8] Iravani S, Korbekandi H, Mirmohammadi SV, Zolfaghari B. Synthesis of silver nanoparticles: Chemical, physical and biological methods. RPS. 2014;**9**(6):385-406

[9] Naseem T, Farrukh MA. Antibacterial activity of green synthesis of iron nanoparticles using *Lawsonia inermis* and *Gardenia jasminoides* leaves extract. Journal of Chemistry. 2015;**912342**

[10] Das VL, Thomas R, Varghese RT, Soniya EV, Mathew J, Radhakrishnan EK. Extracellular synthesis of silver nanoparticles by the *Bacillus* strain CS 11 isolated from industrialized area. 3 Biotech. 2014;**4**(2):121-126

[11] Nanda A, Saravanan M. Biosynthesis of silver nanoparticles from *Staphylococcus aureus* and its antimicrobial activity against MRSA and MRSE. Nanomedicine. 2009;**5**(4):452-456

[12] Shivaji S, Madhu S, Singh S. Extracellular synthesis of antibacterial silver nanoparticles using psychrophilic bacteria. Process Biochemistry. 2011;**49**:830-837

[13] Iravani S. Bacteria in nanoparticle synthesis: Current status and future prospects. International Scholarly Research Notices. Oct 29, 2014;**2014**:359316. DOI: 10.1155/2014/359316

[14] Bagherzade G, Tavakoli MM, Namaei MH. Green synthesis of silver nanoparticles using aqueous extract of saffron (*Crocus sativus* L.) wastages and its antibacterial activity against six bacteria. Asian Pacific Journal of Tropical Biomedicine. 2017;**7**(3):227-233

[15] Raja S, Ramesh V, Thivaharan V. Green biosynthesis of silver nanoparticles using *Calliandra haematocephala* leaf extract, their antibacterial activity and hydrogen peroxide sensing capability. Arabian Journal of Chemistry. 2017;**10**(2):253-261

[16] Verma A, Mehata MS. Controllable synthesis of silver nanoparticles using Neem leaves and their antimicrobial activity. Journal of Radiation Research and Applied Science. 2016;**9**(1):109-115

[17] Patil MP, Singh RD, Koli PB, Patil KT, Jagdale BS, Tipare AR, et al. Antibacterial potential of silver nanoparticles synthesized using *Madhuca longifolia* flower extract as a green resource. Microbial Pathogenesis. 2018;**12**:184-189

[18] Rivera-Rangel RD, González-Muñoz MP, Avila-Rodriguez M, Razo-Lazcano TA, Solans C. Green synthesis of silver nanoparticles in oil-in-water microemulsion and nano-emulsion using geranium leaf aqueous extract as a reducing agent. Colloids and Surfaces A: Physicochemical and Engineering Aspects. 2018;**536**:60-67

[19] Li S, Shen Y, Xie A, Yu X, Qiu L, Zhanga L, et al. Green synthesis of silver nanoparticles using *Capsicum annuum* L. extract. Green Chemistry. 2007;**9**:852-858

[20] Mirgorod YA, Borodina VG. Preparation and bactericidal properties of silver nanoparticles in aqueous tea leaf extract. Inorganic Materials. 2013;**49**(10):980-983

[21] Ahmed S, Ahmad M, Swami BL, Ikram S. A review on plants extract mediated synthesis of silver nanoparticles for antimicrobial applications: A green expertise. Journal of Advanced Research. 2016;**7**(1):17-28

[22] Amin M, Anwar F, Janjua MRSA, Iqbal MA, Rashid U. Green synthesis of silver nanoparticles through reduction with *Solanum xanthocarpum* L. berry extract: Characterization, antimicrobial and urease inhibitory activities against *Helicobacter pylori*. International Journal of Molecular Sciences. 2012;**13**(8):9923-9941

[23] Kim ST, Saha K, Kim C, Rotello VM. The role of surface functionality in determining nanoparticle cytotoxicity. Accounts of Chemical Research. 2013;**46**(3):681-691

[24] Islam NU, Jalil K, Shahid M, Rauf A, Muhammad N, Khan A, et al. Green synthesis and biological activities of gold nanoparticles functionalized with *Salix alba*. Arabian Journal of Chemistry. 2015:12 (in press). DOI: 10.1016/j.arabjc.2015.06.025

[25] Li P, Li S, Wang Y, Zhang Y, Han G. Green synthesis of β-CD-functionalized monodispersed silver nanoparticles with enhanced catalytic activity. Colloids and Surfaces A: Physicochemical and Engineering Aspects. 2017;**520**:26-31

[26] Švecová M, Ulbrich P, Dendisová M, Matějka P. SERS study of riboflavin on green-synthesized silver nanoparticles prepared by reduction using different flavonoids: What is the role of flavonoid used? Spectrochimica Acta. Part A, Molecular and Biomolecular Spectroscopy. 2018;**195**:236-245

[27] Shao Y, Wu C, Wu T, Yuan C, Chen S, Ding T, et al. Green synthesis of sodium alginate-silver nanoparticles and their antibacterial activity. International Journal of Biological Macromolecules. 2018;**111**:1281-1292

[28] Ikram F, Qayoom A, Shah MR. Synthesis of epicatechin coated silver nanoparticles for selective recognition of gentamicin. Sensors and Actuators B: Chemical. 2018;**257**:897-905

[29] Buszewski B, Rafinska K, Pomastowski P, Walczak J, Rogowska A. Novel aspects of silver nanoparticles functionalization. Colloids and Surfaces A: Physicochemical and Engineering Aspects. 2016;**506**:170-178

[30] Kaur A, Goyal D, Kumar R. Surfactant mediated interaction of vancomycin with silver nanoparticles. Applied Surface Science. 2018;**449**:23-30

[31] Sudha A, Jeyakanthan J, Srinivasan P. Green synthesis of silver nanoparticles using *Lippia nodiflora* aerial extract and evaluation of their antioxidant, antibacterial and cytotoxic effects. Resource-Efficient Technologies. 2017;**3**:506-515

[32] Gomathi M, Rajkumar PV, Prakasam A, Ravichandran K. Green synthesis of silver nanoparticles using *Datura stramonium* leaf extract and assessment of their antibacterial activity. Resource-Efficient Technologies. 2017;**3**:280-284

[33] Ahmed KB, Nagy AM, Brown RP, Zhang Q, Malghan SG, Goering PL. Silver nanoparticles: Significance of physicochemical properties and assay interference on the interpretation of in vitro cytotoxicity studies. Toxicology In Vitro. 2017;**38**:179-192

[34] George S, Lin S, Ji Z, Thomas C, Li L, Mecklenburg M, et al. Surface defects on plate-shaped silver nanoparticles contribute to its hazard potential in a fish gill cell line and zebrafish embryos. ACS Nano. 2012;**6**:3745-3759

[35] Kim S, Ryu D. Silver nanoparticle-induced oxidative stress, genotoxicity and apoptosis in cultured cells and animal tissues. Journal of Applied Toxicology. 2013;**33**:78-89

[36] Vedelago J, Gomez CG, Valente M, Mattea F. Green synthesis of silver nanoparticles aimed at improving theranostics. Radiation Physics and Chemistry. 2018;**146**:55-67

[37] Stoehr LC, Gonzalez E, Stampfl A, Casals E, Duschl A, Puntes V, et al. Shape matters: Effects of silver nanospheres and wires on human alveolar epithelial cells. Particle and Fibre Toxicology. 2011;**8**:36

[38] Quinsaat JEQ. Synthesis and functionalization of silver nanoparticles for the preparation of high permittivity nanocomposites [thesis]. Lausanne: EPFL; 2015

[39] Smitha SL, Nissamudeen KM, Philip D, Gopchandran KG. Studies on surface plasmon resonance and photoluminescence of silver nanoparticles. Spectrochimica Acta. Part A, Molecular and Biomolecular Spectroscopy. 2008;**71**:186-190

[40] Castangia I, Marongiu F, Manca ML, Pompei R, Angius F, Ardu A, et al. Combination of grape extract-silver nanoparticles and liposomes: A totally green approach. European Journal of Pharmaceutical Sciences. 2017;**97**:62-69

[41] Azizi S, Mohamad R, Rahim RA, Mohammadinejad R, Ariff AB. Hydrogel beads bio-nanocomposite based on kappa-carrageenan and green synthesized silver nanoparticles for biomedical applications. International Journal of Biological Macromolecules. 2017;**104**:423-431

[42] Zhang X, Servos MR, Liu J. Fast pH-assisted functionalization of silver nanoparticles with monothiolated DNA. Chemical Communications (Cambridge). 2012;**48**(81):10114-10116

[43] Lee J, Lytton-Jean A, Hurst SJ, Mirkin CA. Silver nanoparticle-oligonucleotide conjugates based on DNA with triple cyclic disulfide moieties. Nano Letters. 2007;**7**(7):2112-2115

[44] Prasad SR, Elango K, Damayanthi D, Saranya JS. Formulation and evaluation of azathioprine loaded silver nanopartilces for the treatment of rheumatoid arthritis. AJBPS. 2013;**3**(23):28-32

[45] Dakal TC, Kumar A, Majumdar RS, Yadav V. Mechanistic basis of antimicrobial actions of silver nanoparticles. Frontiers in Microbiology. 2016;**7**:1831

[46] Duran N, Duran M, de Jesus MB, Seabra AB, Favaro WJ, Nakazato G. Silver nanoparticles: A new view on mechanistic aspects on antimicrobial activity. Nanomedicine. 2016;**12**:789-799

[47] Prabhu S, Poulose EK. Silver nanoparticles: Mechanism of antimicrobial action, synthesis, medical applications, and toxicity effects. International Nano Letters. 2012;**2**:32

[48] Abbaszadegan A, Ghahramani Y, Gholami A, Hemmateenejad B, Dorostkar S, Nabavizadeh M, et al. The effect of charge at the surface of silver nanoparticles on antimicrobial activity against gram-positive and gram-negative bacteria: A preliminary study. Journal of Nanomaterials. 2015;**720654**

[49] Keat CL, Aziz A, Eid AM, Elmarzugi NA. Biosynthesis of nanoparticles and silver nanoparticles. Bioresour Bioprocess. 2015;**2**:47

[50] Morones JL, Elichiguerra A, Camacho K, Holt JB, Kouri JT, Ramirez MY. The bactericidal effect of silver nanoparticles. Nanotechnology. 2005;**16**(10):2346-2353

[51] Rai MK, Deshmukh SD, Ingle AP, Gade AK. Silver nanoparticles: The powerful nanoweapon against multidrug-resistant bacteria. Journal of Applied Microbiology. 2012;**112**:841-852

[52] Huang CC, Aronstam RS, Chen D, Huang Y. Oxidative stress, calcium homeostasis and altered gene expression in human lung epithelial cells exposed to ZnO nanoparticles. Toxicology In Vitro. 2010;**24**:45-55

[53] Kvitek L, Panacek A, Soukopova J, Kolar M, Vecerova R, Prucek R, et al. Effect of surfactants and polymers on stability and antibacterial activity of silver nanoparticles (NPs). Journal of Physical Chemistry C. 2008;**112**(15):5825-5834

[54] Pal S, Tak YK, Song JM. Does the antibacterial activity of silver nanoparticles depend on the shape of the nanoparticle? A study of the gram-negative bacterium *Escherichia coli*. Applied and Environmental Microbiology. 2007;**73**(6):1712-1720

[55] Rout A, Jena PK, Sahoo D, Bindhani BK. Green synthesis of silver nanoparticles of different shapes and its antibacterial activity against *Escherichia coli*. International Journal of Current Microbiology and Applied Sciences. 2014;**3**(4):374-383

[56] Sondi I, Salopek-Sondi B. Silver nanoparticles as antimicrobial agent: A case study on *E. coli* as a model from gram-negative bacteria. Journal of Colloid and Interface Science. 2004;**275**(1):177-182

[57] Guzman M, Dille J, Godet S. Synthesis and antibacterial activity of silver nanoparticles against gram-positive and gram-negative bacteria. Nanomedicine. 2012;**8**:37-45

[58] Okafor F, Janen A, Kukhtareva T, Edwards V, Curley M. Green synthesis of silver nanoparticles, their characterization, application and antibacterial activity. International Journal of Environmental Research and Public Health. 2013;**10**:5221-5238

[59] Zhang Y, Yang D, Kong Y, Wang X, Pandoli O, Gao G. Synergetic antibacterial effects of silver nanoparticles @ aloe vera prepared via a green method. Nano Biomedicine and Engineering. 2010;**2**:252-257

[60] Kumar DA, Palanichamy V, Roopan SM. Green synthesis of silver nanoparticles using *Alternanthera dentate* leaf extract at room temperature and their antimicrobial activity. Spectrochimica Acta. Part A, Molecular and Biomolecular Spectroscopy. 2014;**127**: 168-171

[61] Bonde SR, Rathod DP, Ingle AP, Ade RB, Gade AK, Rai MK. *Murraya koenigii*-mediated synthesis of silver nanoparticles and its activity again three human pathogenic bacteria. Journal of Nanoscience Methods. 2012;**1**:25-36

[62] Kajani A, Zarkesh-Esfahani S, Hamid S, Bordbar AK, Khosropour A, Razmjou A, et al. Anticancer effects of silver nanoparticles encapsulated by *Taxus baccata* extracts. Journal of Molecular Liquids. 2016;**223**:549-556

[63] Rao PV, Nallappan D, Madhavi K, Rahman S, Wei LJ, Gan SH. Phytochemical and biogenic metallic nanoparticles as anticancer agents. Oxidative Medicine and Cellular Longevity. 2016;**2016**:3685671. Epub 2016 Feb 23. DOI: 10.1155/2016/3685671

[64] Naz M, Nasiri N, Ikram M, Nafees M, Qureshi MZ, Ali S, et al. Eco-friendly biosynthesis, anticancer drug loading and cytotoxic effect of capped Ag-nanoparticles against breast cancer. Applied Nanoscience. 2017;**7**:793-802

[65] Gurunathan S, Raman J, Abd Malek SN, John PA, Vikineswary S. Green synthesis of silver nanoparticles using Ganoderma neo-japonicum Imazeki: A potential cytotoxic agent against breast cancer cells. International Journal of Nanomedicine. 2013;**8**:4399-4413

[66] Govindaraju K, Krishnamoorthy K, Alsagaby S, Singaravelu G, Premanathan M. Green synthesis of silver nanoparticles for selective toxicity towards cancer cells. IET Nanobiotechnology. 2015;**9**(6):325-330

[67] Salehi S, Shandiz AS, Ghanbar F, Darvish MR, Ardestani M, Mirzaie A, et al. Phytosynthesis of silver nanoparticles using *Artemisia marschalliana* sprengel aerial part extract and assessment of their antioxidant, anticancer, and antibacterial properties. International Journal of Nanomedicine. 2016;**11**:1835-1846

[68] Lakshmanan G, Sathiyaseelan A, Kalaichelvan PT, Murugesan K. Plant-mediated synthesis of silver nanoparticles using fruit extract of *Cleome viscosa* L.: Assessment of their antibacterial and anticancer activity. Karbala International Journal of Modern Science. 2018;**4**:61-68

[69] Singh J, Singh T, Rawat M. Green synthesis of silver nanoparticles via various plant extracts for anti-cancer applications. GJN. 2017;**2**(3). DOI: 1019081/GJN.2017.02.555590

[70] Rath M, Panda SS, Dhal NK. Syntesis of silver nano particles from plant extract and its application in cancer treatment: A review. IJPAES. 2014;**4**(3):137-145

[71] Khalifa KS, Hamouda RA, Hamz HA. Antitumor activity of silver nanoparticles biosynthesized by micro algae. Journal of Chemical and Pharmaceutical Research. 2016;**8**(3):1-6

[72] Gopinath P, Gogoi SK, Chattopadhyay A, Ghosh S. Implications of silver nanoparticle induced cell apoptosis for in vitro gene therapy. Nanotechnology. 2008;**19**(7):075104

[73] Jeyaraj M, Rajesh M, Arun R, MubarakAli D, Sathishkumar G, et al. An investigation on the cytotoxicity and caspase-mediated apoptotic effect of biologically synthesized silver nanoparticles using Podophyllum hexandrum on human cervical carcinoma cells. Colloids and Surfaces. B, Biointerfaces. 2013;**102**:708-717

[74] Blanco MD, Teijón C, Olmo RM, Teijón JM. Targeted nanoparticles for cancer therapy. In: Sezer AD, editor. Recent Advances in Novel Drug Carrier Systems. Rijeka: InTech; 2012. pp. 241-248

[75] Khalid S, Hanif R. Green biosynthesis of silver nanoparticles conjugated to gefitinib as delivery vehicle. IJASET. 2017;**5**(2):59-63

[76] Park W, Na K. Advances in the synthesis and application of nanoparticles for drug delivery. Wiley Interdisciplinary Reviews. Nanomedicine and Nanobiotechnology. 2015;**7**(4):494-508

[77] Brown PK, Qureshi AT, Moll AN, Hayes DJ, Monroe WT. Silver nanoscale antisense drug delivery system for photoactivated gene silencing. ACS Nano. 2013;**7**(4):2948-2959

[78] Qureshi AT. Silver nanoparticles as drug delivery systems [thesis]. Louisiana State University; 2013

[79] Ahamed M, AlSalhi MS, Siddiqui MKJ. Silver nanoparticle applications and human health. Clinica Chimica Acta. 2010;**411**:1841-1848

[80] Braydich-Stolle L, Hussain S, Schlager JJ, Hofmann M-C. In vitro cytotoxicity of nanoparticles in mammalian germline stem cells. Toxicological Sciences. 2005;**88**(2):412-419

[81] Hussain SM, Hess KL, Gearhart JM, Geiss KT, Schlager JJ. In vitro toxicity of nanoparticles in BRL 3A rat liver cells. Toxicology In Vitro. 2005;**19**:975-983

[82] Kim S, Choi JE, Choi J, Chung K-H, Park K, Yi J, et al. Oxidative stress-dependent toxicity of silver nanoparticles in human hepatoma cells. Toxicology In Vitro. 2009;**23**:1076-1084

[83] Singh R, Ramarao P. Cellular uptake, intracellular trafficking and cytotoxicity of silver nanoparticles. Toxicology Letters. 2012;**213**:249-259

[84] Ahamed M, Karns M, Goodson M, Rowe J, Hussain SM, Schlager JJ, et al. DNA damage response to different surface chemistry of silver nanoparticles in mammalian cells. Toxicology and Applied Pharmacology. 2008;**233**:404-410

[85] Beer C, Foldbjerg R, Hayashi Y, Sutherland DS, Autrup H. Toxicity of silver nanoparticles—Nanoparticle or silver ion? Toxicology Letters. 2012;**208**:286-292

[86] Ji JH, Jung JH, Kim SS, Yoon J-Y, Park JD, Choi BS, et al. Twenty-eight-day inhalation toxicity study of silver nanoparticles in Sprague-Dawley rats. Inhalation Toxicology. 2007;**19**:857

[87] Lee H-Y, Choi Y-J, Jung E-J, Yin H-Q, Kwon J-T, Kim J-E, et al. Genomics-based screening of differentially expressed genes in the brains of mice exposed to silver nanoparticles via inhalation. Journal of Nanoparticle Research. 2010;**12**:1567

[88] Kim YS, Kim JS, Cho HS, Rha DS, Kim JM, Park JD, et al. Twenty-eight-day oral toxicity, genotoxicity, and gender-related tissue distribution of silver nanoparticles in Sprague-Dawley rats. Inhalation Toxicology. 2008;**20**:575

Chapter 5

The Role of Natural Dietary Products in Nanomedicine

Heshu Sulaiman Rahman, Hemn Hassan Othman,
Rasedee Abdullah, Nozlena Abdul Smad and
Noorjahan Banu Alitheen

Additional information is available at the end of the chapter

http://dx.doi.org/10.5772/intechopen.79932

Abstract

It has long been established that a diet rich in fresh fruits, vegetables, seeds, grains and legumes and antioxidants, and other beneficial compounds may help prevent various human diseases. However, diet is not a cure for treatment of severe diseases, but it may help prevent some ailments, and it can help the body overcome the effects of conventional treatments. Natural compounds not only serve as a drug or template for drugs but also, in many instances, had been a source of discovery of novel biology that provided better understanding of target and pathway involved in the disease processes. In addition, drugs derived from natural compounds work better for patients than do drugs manufactured synthetically. Approximately, 40% of drugs in the pipeline and 70% of synthetic therapeutic molecules are plagued with poor solubility, oral bioavailability, and delivery. Drugs with poor solubility encounter limited transport during oral administration because of low concentration gradient between the gut and the blood vessels. To increase body fluid saturation solubility of poorly soluble drug, new delivery methods need to be developed using natural dietary plant metabolites.

Keywords: plant metabolite, human ailments, disease therapy, nanomedicine

1. Introduction

1.1. Natural dietary products

Natural product therapeutic compound is a substance or compound produced by living organisms which has pharmacological or biological activity and with potential to be developed into new pharmaceuticals. Natural products may be extracted from plant tissues, marine organisms or microorganism fermentation broths by various mechanical methods [1, 2].

The earliest records of natural products and oldest medical text come from ancient Mesopotamia corresponding to modern-day Iraq (2600 BC), which is written on hundreds of clay tablets in cuneiform. The tablets describe approximately 1000 plants and plant-derived substances, such as the oils of *Cedrus* species (cedar), resin of *Commiphora myrrha* (myrrh), and juice of the poppy seed *Papaver somniferum* with therapeutic potential [3]. The Chinese were the first to use medicinal plants from which over 11,000 herbal remedies were developed and used for thousands of years. In India, natural products are generally accepted as the main disease treatment method, as such almost 70% modern medicines in India are derived from natural products [2].

According to the recent WHO studies, over 30% of plant species of the world have been used for medicinal purposes. Among the estimated 250,000–500,000 higher plant species on earth, more than 80,000 species are purported to possess medicinal properties. However, only a small percentage of these plants has been investigated phytochemically [2]. Some natural compounds are already known to be useful drugs and these include alkaloids, morphine, and quinine, while others such as cocaine have been the basis for synthetic drug development. Among the compound that has been isolated from plants in recent years include the anticancer agent paclitaxel (Taxol) from the yew tree and the antimalarial agent artemisinin from *Artemisia annua* [1].

1.2. Natural products as anticancer agents

It has long been known that a diet rich in fresh fruits, vegetables, seeds, grains, legumes and antioxidants, and other beneficial compounds may help prevent diseases. The evidences are compelling that healthy diet supplemented with vitamins, antioxidants or other beneficial micronutrients has real influence in reducing cancer incidence and mortalities. It was estimated that one-third of all cancer cases could be prevented by a healthy diet [4, 5].

Although the search for natural compounds against cancers is still ongoing and exhaustive, more than 100 new products have already been developed for cancer therapy. However, the potential discovery of new cancer therapeutics is still enormous because approximately 80% of the rain forest plant species are likely to contain chemicals with anticancer properties, while only a fraction of these plants has been analyzed for their therapeutic properties [6].

There are several compounds from natural products that can directly or indirectly serve to treat cancers. The immune system can be boosted to recognize cancer cells through glutamine, melatonin, parthenolide, resveratrol (from red grape), carotenoids (pigments in vegetables), indole-3-carbinol, vitamin D, emodin, vitamin E, genistein (from red clover and soy products), proanthocyanides (from grape seed and pine bark), flavonoids (from tea family and berry family), and lycopene (from tomatoes) [7]. Other compounds proposed to have anticancer properties are garlic (*Allium sativum*), ginkgo (*Ginkgo biloba*), echinacea (*Echinacea purpurea*), ginseng (*Panax ginseng*), St John's wort (*Hypericum perforatum*), ginger (*Zingiber zerumbet*), kava (*Piper methysticum*) [8] and cabbage, licorice, onions, flax, turmeric, cruciferous vegetables, peppers, brown rice, wheat, and the umbelliferous vegetables such as carrots, celery, and parsley [6].

http://dx.doi.org/10.5772/intechopen.79932

1.2.1. Zingiber

Ginger herb with white, red, or yellow flowers and dark green leaves and thick roots is a set of plants with various medicinal and culinary values found in many parts of the world including Malaysia. Ginger belongs to the genus *Zingiber* representing approximately 141 species under the family Zingiberaceae. The word ginger comes from the Latin Sanskrit word Sringavera, meaning that the rhizomes look like antlers of deer or horns of bull. The underground stems of ginger, which is the rhizomes, are knobby and fleshy, covered in ring-like scars and are used as food and medicine. Among the ginger, species with potential for high medicinal values are *Zingiber officinale* and *Zingiber zerumbet* [8, 9].

1.2.2. Zingiber zerumbet (L.) Smith

Zingiber zerumbet (L.) Smith (**Figure 1**) is an edible ginger, native to India and the Malay Peninsula, although it can be found in many countries including Indonesia, China, Bangladesh, Vietnam, Japan, Burma, Nepal, Sri Lanka, Jamaica, and Nigeria. This herbal plant is commonly known as the pinecone, wild ginger, Asian ginger or shampoo ginger. It is known by various names in different countries such as *lempoyang* in Malaysia and Indonesia, *Ghatian* and *Yaiimu* in India, *Jangliadah* in Bangladesh, *Hong qui jiang* in China, *Haeo dam* in Northern Thailand, *Awapuhi* in Hawaii, and *zurunbah* among the Arabians [8]. Generally, the rhizomes and leaves are used for spice, tea, beverages, and medical purposes, while the milky, mucilaginous substance of the pinecones is used as shampoo and natural hair conditioner [9].

Zingiber zerumbet contains several types of phytochemicals and is considered as one of the widely used traditional dietary condiments for cuisines, food, and beverages throughout the Asia, and the essential oil is used as perfume and toilet article. In traditional oriental medicine, the oil is used for a variety of digestive conditions [10]. The extract of the rhizome has been extensively studied for its antimicrobial, anticonvulsant, antipyretic, analgesic, antiulcer, antioxidant, antitumor, anticancer, antispasmodic, anti-inflammatory, antinociceptive, anticoagulant, antidiabetic, antihyperlipidemic and antiobesogenic, antiallergenic, anti-platelet aggregation, and hepatoprotective activities. Additional studies

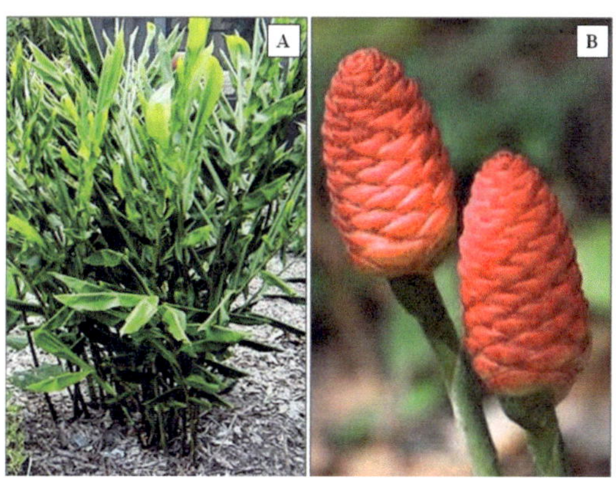

Figure 1. *Zingiber zerumbet* (A) tree and (B) inflorescence.

had showed that rhizome consumption can lower blood cholesterol levels by reducing cholesterol absorption in the blood and liver, making this extract useful for treatment of heart diseases [11–13].

1.2.3. Ginger oil

Ginger oil is obtained from unpeeled or dried, ground-up root (rhizome) of *Zingiber zerumbet* by steam distillation. Ginger oil can vary in color from pale yellow to a dark amber, and the viscosity ranges from medium to watery. It has a strong spicy odor, sharp, warm and with a hint of lemon and pepper, and smells of actual ginger. The taste of ginger oil is peculiar and pungent [14].

1.2.4. Zerumbone

Zerumbone (ZER) was first isolated in 1960 from the essential volatile oil of rhizomes of *Zingiber zerumbet*, while its structure was first determined in 1965 and later characterized by NMR and X-ray. Zerumbone (**Figure 2**) is a sesquiterpene phytochemical compound isolated from *Zingiber zerumbet* (L.) smith or *Zingiber aromaticum*. It contains three double bonds, two conjugated and one isolated, as well as a conjugated carbonyl group in 11-membrane ring structure [16, 17]. Among parts of the plant richest in ZER are rhizomes followed by the leaves [18, 19]. Zerumbone is also the major compound (59%) in the essential oil from *Zingiber zerumbet* [20].

1.3. General medicinal properties of zerumbone

Several biological activities of ZER have been reported both *in vivo* and *in vitro*. These studies have found ZER to possess antitumor, anti-inflammatory, antioxidant, antimicrobial, antinociceptive, antiatherosclerosis, hepatoprotective, antiplatelet aggregation, and immunomodulatory activities at different doses and concentrations [21].

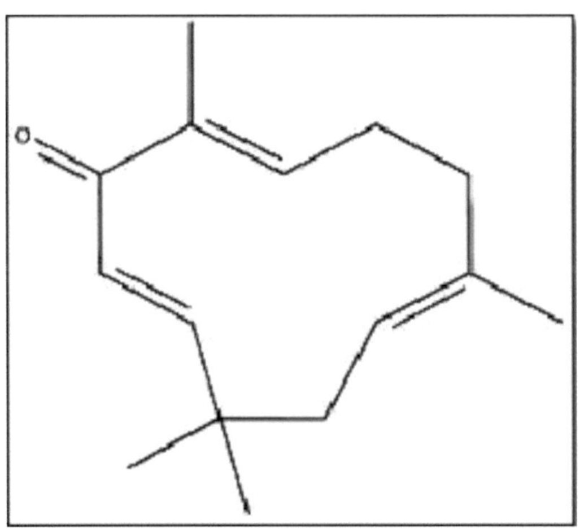

Figure 2. Chemical structure of zerumbone [15].

1.4. Carrier systems for drug delivery

Generally, the number of drugs and drug candidates is steadily increasing over the last 2 decades. A number of these drugs have poor water solubility, which consequently cause poor oral bioavailability and delivery. Drug of poor bioavailability will not be readily absorbed from the gastrointestinal tract into circulation and would not reach the site of action. However, solubilization of poorly soluble drugs is limited by drug properties, chemistry, molecular size, and selective solubility in certain organic media [22]. For several year approaches to increase drug solubility by solubilization with surfactants, complex formation (cyclodextrins and macromolecules), microemulsions, and micronization of drug powders to increase the surface area and stability has not been very successful because the dissolution velocity of these drug was insufficient to overcome the lack of bioavailability to meet biopharmaceutical specification [23]. Therefore, there is a desperate need to develop innovative pharmaceutical carriers and delivery systems that overcome these drawbacks. Generally, carrier schemes for drug delivery should be toxicity-free, possess sufficient drug loading capacity, and have tissue targeting and controlled release characteristics. The carriers should also afford chemical and physical stability to incorporated drug. To achieve their commercial potentials, these carrier and delivery systems should be feasible for production scaling-up at reasonable costs [24].

1.5. Colloidal carrier system

Colloidal drug carrier systems (**Figure 3**) have received great attention as potential drug delivery system because they offer many advantages as drug delivery vehicles including capability of increasing dissolution velocity that also increases bioavailability and solubility saturation. This can be achieved by reducing the size of the particle that increases surface area while increasing dissolution velocity. Thus, suitable nanoparticles can be employed as delivery systems with solid colloidal particle size ranging from 1 to 1000 nm [25].

Colloids consist of least two components; one dispersed in the other as fine particles in any state of matter. As pharmaceutical carriers, colloidal drug delivery systems can be classed into polymer systems (micelles, dendrimers, etc.), self-assembled lipid systems (liposomes, emulsions, SLN, NLC, etc.), drug nanoparticle systems, and pro-colloidal systems (self-emulsifying oral delivery systems and liquid crystalline systems) [23]. Lipids are physiologically natural occurring compounds that are well tolerated, usually nontoxic or degradable to nontoxic residues. Thus, the lipid-based nanoparticles provide an advantage over other types of carrier systems. Liposomes and micelles are among the first colloidal drug carriers developed to overcome the possibilities of water-insoluble drug formulations [26]. They are naturally derived phospholipids and surfactant vesicles that can be filled with various drugs [27]. Liposomes and micelles are rapidly degradation by the pH of the stomach, intestinal enzymes, and bile salts after oral administration but have restricted physical and chemical stability during storage. These particles characteristically cause fast release of the drug while not so stable over extended period of storage. The liposomes and micelles also leave behind residues of the organic solvents and cause some degrees of toxicity to normal tissues. These characteristics make these colloidal carriers not optimal as a pharmaceutical carrier system.

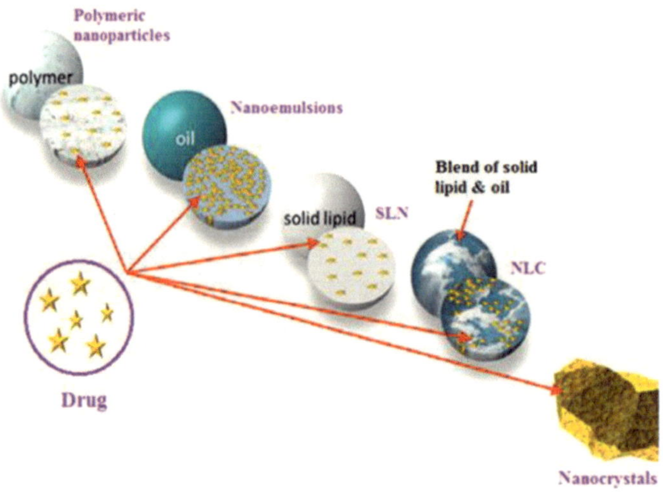

Figure 3. Various types of nanoparticles as drug delivery system. SLN—solid lipid nanoparticle and NLC—nanostructured lipid carrier. (http://www.pharmatutor.org/articles/nanotechnology-nanocrystal, 2013).

1.6. Nanoparticles

Solid lipid nanoparticle (SLN) (**Figure 4**) is also a colloidal drug carrier system developed as an alternative system to the existing traditional carrier systems [28]. Although SLN have numerous advantages including targeted drug delivery and increased stability of incorporated drug, they are still fraught with limitations. The matrix of SLN is highly ordered crystalline lipid structure leaving very little space for incorporation of drug molecules, thus limiting the loading capacity. The net effect of these properties is expulsion of incorporated during storage. To overcome these limitations, a second generation lipid nanoparticle, the nanostructured lipid carrier (NLC) was introduced [29]. Nanostructured lipid carrier is a novel lipid nanoparticle, which in contrast to SLN consists of a mixture of solid and liquid lipids, in fine proportions. This formulation of NLC prevents the formation of perfect crystals and minimizes the drug expulsion phenomenon during storage [30]. With the introduction of NLC, lipid colloid carriers began to gain new life as a potential drug carrier and delivery system [29].

In last couple of years, NLC has attracted great attention as an alternate carrier for the pharmaceutical for anticancer drugs [24]. The NLC contains liquid lipids with different fatty acid C-chains responsible for producing the less-organized crystalline structure, providing better and higher drug loading capacity accommodation [31]. Several methods have been used to prepare the lipid nanoparticles of different size, surface characteristic, and stability. The preparation of stable NLC of high surface area is based on three principles, namely precipitation, milling, and high pressure homogenization [22]. In the precipitation phase, the drug is dissolved in a solvent and subsequently added to a nanosolvent resulting in the precipitation of finely dispersed drug nanoparticles [25]. In the milling method, the dimension of particles is achieved by using different sizes of bead, ball mills or a pearl mill that consisting of ceramics, stainless steel, glass or highly cross linked polystyrene resin coated as milling media. The high pressure homogenization (HPH) generates small nanoparticle under pressure. Surfactants are required to stabilize the particle at the desired size. Lipid nanoparticles can also be produced by either hot or cold HPH technique. Other less common methods include spray drying,

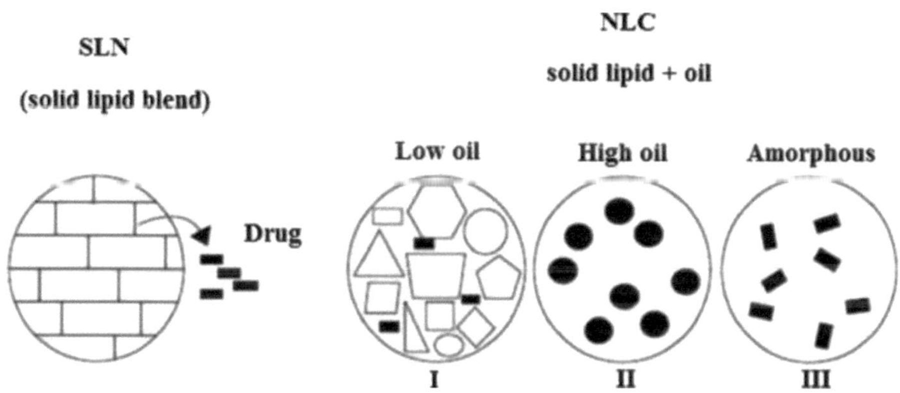

Figure 4. Solid lipid nanoparticle and nanostructured lipid carriers. I—highly imperfect matrix, II—multiple oil/fat/water type, and III—noncrystalline nanostructured nanoparticle [24].

ultrasonication, solvent evaporation, film ultrasound dispersion, microemulsion based, and supercritical fluid methods [25].

1.7. Nanostructured lipid carriers

Nanostructured lipid carriers are fine blends between solid and liquid lipids stabilized by the introduction of surfactants. Three different approaches have been developed to optimize the structure of NLC. First, imperfect type or type I NLC is prepared by blending spatially different lipid types (solid and oil) to create distance between the fatty acid chains of the glycerides and imperfections in the crystal. This procedure offers more space for the accommodation of drug molecules and amorphous clusters of drugs, thus higher drug loading in the NLC. At the final stage, solid particles are produced by crystallization of liquid lipid particles (nanoemulsions) at room temperature from the cooled molten state. Basically, drug solubility is higher in liquid lipids than in solid lipids, and thus particles produced with high content of liquid lipids can load more drug [32]. Multiple type or type II NLC is prepared by mixing high liquid lipid, solid lipid, water, and drug. The high oil concentrations produce miscibility gap between solid lipids and liquid lipids during the cooling phase leading to phase separation and consequently precipitation of tiny oily nanocompartments. Finally, amorphous type or type III or multiple oil/fat/water type NLC is prepared by mixing solid lipids while in amorphous state. Solid lipid particle crystallization that can occur upon cooling is prevented by adding special lipids such as hydroxyoctacosanyl-hydroxystearate and isopropyl myristate [25, 32].

1.8. Characterization of nanostructured lipid carriers

Characterization of NLC is essential to determine the properties of the nanoparticle. Among the techniques employed to characterize nanoparticles include image analysis which includes light microscope, scanning electron microscope (SEM), transmission electron microscope (TEM), and atomic force microscope (AFM) to characterize and determine particle size and shape. Nuclear magnetic resonance (NMR) is used to determine particle size and qualitative nature of nanoparticle. Other characteristics of nanoparticles of concern are zeta potential (ZP), which characterizes ionization properties that dictates the agglomeration behavior of nanoparticles. Polydispersity index (PDI) is a measure of distribution of molecular mass in a given polymer sample. It is a measure of particle size distribution. The PDI values are always greater than 1; however, as the size becomes more uniform, the PDI approaches 1. The ZP, PDI, and particle can be determined using a Zetasizer. The efficiency of nanoparticles as a drug carrier system can be partially determined by the entrapment efficiency (EE) and drug loading (DL) capacity. Entrapment efficiency is the ratio of weight of drug entrapped in a carrier system to the total drug added, while DL is the ratio of drug to the weight of the total carrier system. The EE and DL can be determined by high performance liquid chromatography (HPLC) technique, which at the same time can be used to determine the content of a substance and/or its chemical stability. It is optimal for a drug delivery system to exhibit sustained release characteristics. This feature of drug-loaded nanoparticles can be analyzed using the Franz Diffusion Cell (FDC), which determines the rate of drug release from lipid particles. Thermal stability is another important feature of a drug carrier and nanoparticle delivery systems. This is essential because the preparation of these particles is done under high temperatures. The differential scanning calorimetry (DSC) is used to determine the physical and energetic properties of a substance as a function of temperature. The X-ray diffractometer was developed to measure the geometric scattering radiation from crystal planes within nanoparticle dispersion for assessing the degree of crystallinity using wide-angle X-ray diffraction (WXRD) [33, 34].

1.9. Nanoparticles in parenteral applications

In disease therapy, nanoparticles can be administered via several routes of administration, that is, parenteral, oral, intraocular, rectal, nasal, transdermal, or pulmonary inhalation [25, 35]. Thus, the understanding of the nature of targets and their interaction of the nanoparticles in a biological environment is imperative in the design of carrier systems [33]. Nanoparticles are large enough to be removed from circulation after intravenous injection by the macrophages through phagocytosis. Thus, this rapid removal of colloidal particles by the free circulating macrophages is a major obstacle of tissue targeting of drug-loaded nanoparticles. Similarly, fixed macrophages in tissue can also be phagocytose carrier drugs. Particles smaller than 7 μm are normally trapped in the small pulmonary vessels, while larger particles will pass through capillary beds of lungs to liver and spleen, which are then engulfed by the fixed macrophages. Consequently, these organs will be the primary deposition sites for small nanoparticles [32]. The size, surface properties of carrier, and the total amount of serum protein adsorbed on the surface of nanoparticle are the most important factors affecting the macrophage uptake process of drug carrier. The rate of clearance of the drug carriers is approximately proportional to the amount of serum protein adsorbed on their surfaces. Hydrophobic particles will be removed from the circulation more rapidly than hydrophilic particles. Thus, to prolong circulation time, the drug carrier should be formulated with little to no serum adsorption. Currently, among the challenges is the design and formulation of colloidal carriers with prolonged distribution in the body is to find means to delay clearance from the body by avoiding the macrophages of the monocyte-phagocytic system [25].

1.10. Nanoparticles for cancer therapy

The development of nanotechnology is exponential and touted to be the technology that could revolutionize how drugs are delivered. Transfer of materials into the nanodimensions changes their physical properties but not their biological activities, and this phenomenon is used in pharmaceutics to develop new innovative formulations for poorly soluble drugs [36]. The use of nanotechnology in cancer treatment offers some exciting possibilities, including tissue targeting and destruction of cancerous cells and tumors with minimal toxicity to the healthy tissue and organs. If well designed, the formulations may detect and eliminate cancer cells early before they form tumors [37]. The small size of nanoparticles endows them with properties that allow them to preferentially accumulate at tumor sites and when used in association with magnetic resonance imaging (MRI) can produce exceptional images of the tumors. Another property of nanoparticles is the high surface area to volume ratio that allows many functional groups to be attached, for example, groups that can seek out and bind to tumor cells [38].

2. Conclusion

Cancer nanotherapeutics is rapidly progressing and is being implemented to overcome limitations of conventional drug delivery systems. Early clinical results suggest that nanoparticle therapeutics shows enhanced efficacy, while reducing side effects. The major role of nanoparticle in drug delivery is to increase the dissolution velocity by reduction size and increasing surface area and bioavailability. Nanoparticle can carry loaded drugs to cancer cells selectively through the unique pathophysiology of tumors, such as enhanced permeability and retention of drugs in the tumor microenvironment.

Author details

Heshu Sulaiman Rahman[1,2]*, Hemn Hassan Othman[3,4], Rasedee Abdullah[5], Nozlena Abdul Smad[6] and Noorjahan Banu Alitheen[1,7]

*Address all correspondence to: heshu.rhaman@univsul.edu.my

1 Department of Cell and Molecular Biology, Faculty of Biotechnology and Biomolecular Sciences, Universiti Putra Malaysia, Selangor, Malaysia

2 Department of Clinic and Internal Medicine, College of Veterinary Medicine, University of Sulaimani, Sulaimani City, Kurdistan Region, Republic of Iraq

3 Department of Histology and Anatomy, College of Veterinary Medicine, University of Sulaimani, Sulaimani City, Kurdistan Region, Republic of Iraq

4 Department of Pathology and Microbiology, Faculty of Veterinary Medicine, Universiti Putra Malaysia, Selangor, Malaysia

5 Department of Veterinary Laboratory Diagnosis, Faculty of Veterinary Medicine, Universiti Putra Malaysia, Selangor, Malaysia

6 Integrative Medicine Cluster, Advanced Medical and Dental Institute, Universiti Sains Malaysia, Kepala Batas, Penang, Malaysia

7 Institute of Bioscience, Universiti Putra Malaysia, Selangor, Malaysia

References

[1] Brahmachari G. Natural Products in Drug Discovery: Impacts and Opportunities—An Assessment. Singapore: World Scientific Publishing Company; 2011. pp. 1-199

[2] Srujana TS, Babu KR, Rao BSS. Phytochemical investigation and biological activity of leaves extract of plant Boswellia Serrata. The Pharma Innovation. 2012;**1**:25-52

[3] Dias DA, Urban S, Roessner U. A Historical Overview of Natural Products in Drug Discovery. Metabolites. 2012;**2**(2):303-336

[4] Freedman ND, Cross AJ, Mcglynn KA, Abnet CC, Park Y, Hollenbeck AR, et al. Association of meat and fat intake with liver disease and hepatocellular carcinoma in the NIH-AARP cohort. Journal of the National Cancer Institute. 2010;**102**:1354-1365

[5] Wicki A, Hagmann J. Diet and cancer. Swiss Medical Weekly. 2011;**141**:13250

[6] Pan MH, Ho CT. Chemopreventive effects of natural dietary compounds on cancer development. Chemical Society Reviews. 2008;**37**:2558-2574

[7] Muriel JM. Herbs or natural products that decrease cancer growth. Oncology Nursing Forum. 2004;**31**

[8] Yob N, Jofrry SM, Affandi M, Teh L, Salleh M, Zakaria Z. *Zingiber zerumbet* (L.) Smith: A review of its ethnomedicinal, chemical, and pharmacological uses. Evidence-based Complementary and Alternative Medicine. 2011

[9] Basak S, Sarma GC, Rangan L. Ethnomedical uses of Zingiberaceous plants of Northeast India. Journal of Ethnopharmacology. 2010;**132**:286-296

[10] Prakash RO, Rabinarayan A, Kumar MS. *Zingiber zerumbet* (L.) Sm., a reservoir plant for therapeutic uses: A review. International Journal of Research in Ayurveda and Pharmacy. 2011;**2**:1-22

[11] Chang CJ, Tzeng TF, Liou SS, Chang YS, Liu IM. Regulation of lipid disorders by ethanol extracts from *Zingiber zerumbet* in high-fat diet-induced rats. Food Chemistry. 2012; **132**:460-467

[12] Tzeng TF, Liou SS, Chang CJ, Liu IM. The ethanol extract of *Zingiber zerumbet* attenuates streptozotocin-induced diabetic nephropathy in rats. Evidence-based Complementary and Alternative Medicine. 2013

[13] Tzeng TF, Liu IM. 6-Gingerol prevents adipogenesis and the accumulation of cytoplasmic lipid droplets in 3T3-L1 cells. Phytomedicine. 2013

[14] Takada Y, Murakami A, Aggarwal BB. Zerumbone abolishes NF-kappaB and IkappaB alpha kinase activation leading to suppression of antiapoptotic and metastatic gene expression, upregulation of apoptosis, and downregulation of invasion. Oncogene. 2005;**24**:6957-6969

[15] Abdelwahab SI, Abdul AB, Devi N, Ehassan Taha MM, Al-Zubairi AS, Mohan S, et al. Regression of cervical intraepithelial neoplasia by zerumbone in female Balb/c mice prenatally exposed to diethylstilboestrol: Involvement of mitochondria-regulated apoptosis. Experimental and Toxicologic Pathology. 2010;**62**:461-469

[16] Kitayama T, Yokoi T, Kawai Y, Hill RK, Morita M, Okamoto T, et al. The chemistry of zerumbone. Part 5: Structural transformation of the dimethylamine derivatives. Tetrahedron. 2003;**59**:4857-4866

[17] Kitayama T, Furuya A, Moriyama C, Masuda T, Fushimi S, Yonekura Y, et al. Elucidation of the sharpless epoxidation of zerumbol. Tetrahedron: Asymmetry. 2006;**17**:2311-2316

[18] Bhuiyan MNI, Chowdhury JU, Begum J. Chemical investigation of the leaf and rhizome essential oils of *Zingiber zerumbet* (L.) Smith from Bangladesh. Bangladesh Journal of Pharmacology. 2008;**4**:9-12

[19] Chane-Ming J, Vera R, Chalchat JC. Chemical composition of the essential oil from rhizomes, leaves and flowers of *Zingiber zerumbet* Smith from Reunion Island. Journal of Essential Oil Research. 2003;**15**:202-205

[20] Duve R. Highlights of the chemistry and pharmacology of wild ginger (*Zingiber zerumbet* Smith). Fiji Agricultural Journal. 1980;**42**:41-43

[21] Somchit MN, Mak JH, Ahmad Bustamam A, Zuraini A, Arifah AK, Adam Y, et al. Zerumbone isolated from *Zingiber zerumbet* inhibits inflammation and pain in rats. Journal of Medicinal Plant Research. 2012;**6**:177-180

[22] Junghanns JH, Müller RH. Nanocrystal technology, drug delivery and clinical applications. International Journal of Nanomedicine. 2008;**3**:295-309

[23] Sahu MK, Soni GC, Prajapati SK. Formulation and characterization of topical nanostructured lipid carrier gel of Flurbiprofen and its composition with micellar gel preparation. World Journal of Pharmaceutical Sciences. 2012;**1**:1235-1247

[24] Selvamuthukumar S, Velmurugan R. Nanostructured lipid carriers: A potential drug carrier for cancer chemotherapy. Lipids in Health and Disease. 2012;**11**:1-8

[25] Ekambaram P, Sathali AH, Priyanka K. Solid lipid nanoparticles: A review. Scientific Reviews and Chemical Communications. 2012;**2**:80-102

[26] Gregoriadis G. Liposomes as Drug Carriers: Recent Trends and Progress. Wiley Chichester; 1988

[27] Gomez-Hens A, Fernandez-Romero J. Analytical methods for the control of liposomal delivery systems. TrAC Trends in Analytical Chemistry. 2006;**25**:167-178

[28] Pawar BB, Gavale CS. Solid lipid nanoparticles: The beneficial carrier for the delivery of lipid soluble drugs. International Journal of Periodontics and Restorative Dentistry. 2012;**3**:200-209

[29] Meghana SK, Krunal KV, Ashok VB, Pravin DC. Solid lipid nanoparticles and nanostructured lipid carriers. International Journal of Pharma and Bio Sciences. 2012;**2**:681-691

[30] Fathi M, Varshosaz J, Mohebbi M, Shahidi F. Hesperetin-loaded solid lipid nanoparticles and nanostructure lipid carriers for food fortification: Preparation, characterization, and modeling. Food and Bioprocess Technology. 2012:1-12

[31] Yuechao D. Fabrication and characterization of low crystalline curcumin loaded lipid nanoparticles [MSc thesis]. New Brunswick, USA: University of New Jersey; 2011

[32] Akhayachatra C. Development of lipid nanoparticles for anticancer drug delivery systems [PhD thesis]. Thailand: Silpakorn University; 2009

[33] Dubey A, Prabhu P, Kamath JV. Nano structured lipid carriers: A novel topical drug delivery system. International Journal of PharmTech Research. 2012;**4**:705-714

[34] Nam SH, Ji XY, Park JS. Investigation of tacrolimus loaded nanostructured lipid carriers for topical drug delivery. Bulletin of the Korean Chemical Society. 2011;**32**:956-960

[35] Mulla AS, Shetty NS, Panchamukhi SI, Khazi IA. Formulation, characterization and in vitro evaluation of novel thienopyrimidies and triazolothienopyrimidies loaded solid lipid nanoparticles. International Journal of Research in Ayurveda and Pharmacy. 2010; **1**:192-200

[36] Tiwari M. Nano cancer therapy strategies. Journal of Cancer Research and Therapeutics. 2012;**8**:19

[37] Mathur V, Satrawala Y, Rajput MS, Kumar P, Shrivastava P, Vishvkarma A. Solid lipid nanoparticles in cancer therapy. International Journal of Drug Delivery. 2011;**2**

[38] Duncan R. The dawning era of polymer therapeutics. Nature Reviews Drug Discovery. 2003;**2**:347-360